Por

SYBILLA AVERY COOK

Second Edition

 Endorsed by the American Volkssport Association

FALCON GUIDES

GUILFORD, CONNECTICUT
HELENA, MONTANA

AN IMPRINT OF GLOBE PEQUOT PRESS

To buy books in quantity for corporate use
or incentives, call **(800) 962-0973**
or e-mail **premiums@GlobePequot.com**.

FALCON GUIDES®

Unless otherwise noted, all photos are by Sybilla Avery Cook.

Text design: Elizabeth Kingsbury
Layout artist: Kirsten Livingston
Project editor: Ellen Urban

Maps by Trailhead Graphics, Inc. © Morris Book Publishing, LLC

Library of Congress Cataloging-in-Publication Data is available on file.

ISBN 978-0-7627-7806-5

Printed in the United States of America

10 9 8 7 6 5 4 3 2

To Carolyn and Bob Cook, who checked facts and walks, found interesting places, and gave needed and varied support.

Contents

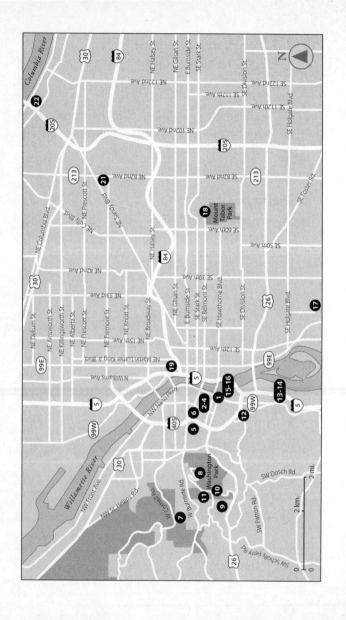

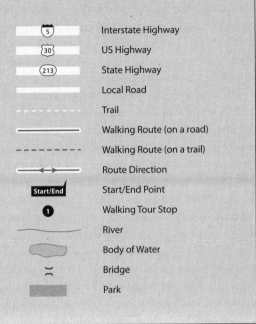

Map Legend

	Interstate Highway
	US Highway
	State Highway
	Local Road
	Trail
	Walking Route (on a road)
	Walking Route (on a trail)
	Route Direction
Start/End	Start/End Point
1	Walking Tour Stop
	River
	Body of Water
	Bridge
	Park

Acknowledgments

This could not have been written without the help of many wonderful people. First and foremost are my sons Bob and Hal, daughter-in-law Carolyn, and grandchildren Matt and Avery Cook, who provided information, companionship, and technical support.

It proved invaluable to re-walk Portland in the company of knowledgeable and enthusiastic Portland residents. I could not have managed this project without them. Dick and Dot Lukins not only provided excellent company, but Dick also took countless photographs to illustrate the book and provide memory checks. Bernadette Crepau, Jeanne Webb, Diana Harris, and Gary Piercy not only cheered me on, but they also showed (and told) me about some of their favorite places. Authors Stephen Leflar (*A History of South Portland*) and Tracy J. Prince (*Portland's Goose Hollow*) generously guided me to some of their favorite discoveries. Eric Kimmel found time between writing his picture books and teaching abroad to take me around the Beverly Cleary neighborhood. Cleary's children's books and autobiographies had made Portland seem like a friendly place long before I managed to see it for myself.

Mary Ellen Marmaduke is one of the countless people who have filled me in on Portland's everyday history. She encouraged me, assisted with research, proofread pages, and made suggestions to ensure that the South Portland walks were both accurate and interesting. She introduced me to many citizens who are constantly working to keep Portland the wonderful city it is, from designing parks to historic preservation. Doug Macy, one of the landscape architects who has created many of Portland's new urban designs, answered many questions. Gloria Catalan has lived in South Portland since childhood; her stories helped bring the neighborhood to life, as did those of Ardyth Shapiro, Mary Bosch, Jacquie Lung, and many others. Don and Mary Louise Sevetson, Mary Zehrung, Ottomar Rudolf, Susan Marmaduke, Patti Gazely, and Bob Clay showed me through their neighborhoods, pointing out things of interest I might have overlooked. Rolf Glerum's Portland knowledge and research skills proved invaluable. Janice Dilg and her Portland State University students added their knowledge of women's contributions to Portland history. The Mirabella Portland retirement community staff also shared their knowledge of the city, and willingly managed my many odd demands.

Jenica Cogdill, Jeanette Hansen, Joan McCoy, Sara McCausland, and Suzanne Walker also volunteered their time as fact-checkers. They re-walked the routes to make sure the directions were clear and would work. Their thorough notes and corrections were invaluable.

Heather Bayles, Tom Costello, Darcy Cronis, Marci Cochran, Pam England, Martin Nicholson, Mark Ross, and Bill Zanze, among others, have patiently answered many questions about parks, art, plants, and fountains. They represent many city employees and volunteers whose enthusiasm about the city and their work makes this a wonderful place to live and visit.

Preface: Come Walk Portland

*Look up. Look down. Look all around
to see the sights in Portland Town.*

Each time I walk through Portland this bit of rhyme runs through my head. Interesting signs, architectural details, and an eclectic assortment of art pieces are overhead, on every side, and etched in the sidewalks underfoot. These unexpected touches add to the charm of walking through the city.

Since the publishing of this book fifteen years ago, Portland remains the same beautiful, livable, and progressive city. Some things have changed, but the features that made the city so appealing are still present. Tucked between the Pacific Ocean and the Cascade Range at the confluence of the Columbia and Willamette Rivers, Portland delights walkers with its natural beauty. The seafarers and merchants who founded this port city were experienced travelers. Having enjoyed the parks and plazas of the world's loveliest cities, they created a community that included grassy sanctuaries within this City of Roses. In spite of all the rain jokes, the city's generally mild weather is a boon to walkers. "Rainy" days are often only misty, and sunny summer days are among Portland's best-kept secrets.

Portland was founded in 1845, but fire or flood destroyed most of the early wooden buildings. Elegant and architecturally interesting turn-of-the-century structures replaced them. As you amble through the city, you will pass many graceful old mansions and walk through neighborhoods that embody what was then state-of-the-art planning. Snowcapped Mount Hood and Mount St. Helens form the backdrop to parks, forests, sloughs, the Willamette River waterfront, and Portland's world-famous roses.

This is a city constantly renewing itself. I have been amazed at the new artwork, the old works that seem to move locations overnight, and the once-neglected homes that are now charming. A worldlier city has evolved, with more high-rises, public transportation, and increased emphasis on being environmentally sound. The rain and concerned citizens have kept Portland beautiful; citizens still buy print books in local bookstores; and "craft" beers have put Portland on the map. Builders now strive for high LEED (Leadership in Energy and Environmental Design) ratings. As the Willamette runs cleaner, more activities are centered on and beside it, and on the new Esplanade that allows runners, walkers, and bike riders to circle the river.

Other signs of the times: The Portland Streetcar system is new with two lines (North-South and Central Loop) connecting with the MAX lines at Pioneer Square. There are more bicycles and bike lanes, and more hybrid and electric cars. OHSU (Oregon Health and Science University) ran out of space on Marquam Hill and has expanded to the newly developed South Waterfront, with its Center for Health and Healing for outpatient services. A new dental school plus medical and research buildings are being constructed on the Schnitzer campus north of the Ross Island Bridge. South of this bridge is Portland's newest neighborhood, South Waterfront, with high-rise condos, apartments, parks, and street-level restaurants and services.

An overhead tram connects both areas, and a pedestrian bridge spanning eleven lanes of freeway connects to the west side.

Some tastes have changed. The beloved baseball team, the Portland Beavers, left Civic Stadium for another town; and the Portland Timbers, a major league soccer team, now occupies the newly named Jeld-Wen Field. On the east side the Portland Trail Blazers still play in the Rose Garden, along with the Winterhawks ice hockey team. Portlanders love both active and spectator sports.

From almost the very beginning, the city has been graced by outstanding building and landscape architects. A. E. Doyle and Associates, inspired by the "White City" of the 1893 World's Columbian Exposition, designed many classic downtown buildings that were clad in white-glazed terra-cotta. They now form a historically significant collection. Italian architectural engineer Pietro Belluschi received an advanced engineering degree from Cornell University and worked in Doyle's firm. His Pacific Northwest Regional designs and use of wood also grace the city. As you walk by these buildings, you can see how well his works blend with a variety of surroundings.

The park plans of the Olmsted Brothers have been copied and adjusted to accommodate the changing times, but they are still beautiful and well used. Modernist Lawrence Halprin and later landscape architects have designed more urban parks as the city has grown. Halprin's Keller Fountain exemplifies his desire to make holistic and varied spaces where people can visit, play, and live. Walker Macy's Vietnam Veterans Memorial and Portland University Transit Center, along with Mayer/Reed's Esplanade, are a few examples of other modern landscape designs that will continue to enhance the city in the future.

If you live in Oregon, *Walking Portland* will give you and your visitors a taste of what makes Portland special. If you are in Portland for business or pleasure, you will find stress-free getaways within walking distance of your hotel. From forest trails to waterfront promenades, Portland offers business travelers, tourists, and residents many miles of enjoyable walking.

Introduction

Walking a city's boulevards and avenues can take you into its heart and give you a feel for its pulse and personality. Looking up from the sidewalk, you can appreciate a city's architecture. Peering in from the sidewalk, you can find the quaint shops, local museums, and great eateries that give a city its charm and personality. From a city's nature paths, you can smell the flowers, glimpse the wildlife, gaze at a lake, or hear a creek gurgle, and only from the sidewalk can you get close enough to read the historical plaques and watch the people.

When you walk a city, you get it all: adventure, scenery, local color, good exercise, and fun.

How to Use This Guide

To easily find the walks that match your interests, time, and energy level, start with the Trip Planner. This table will give you the basic information—a walk's distance, estimated walking time, and difficulty. The pictures or icons in the table will also tell you specific things about the walk. Here is what those icons mean:

📷 If you like to take pictures, then you will get some scenic shots or vistas on this walk. Every walk has something of interest, but this icon tells you that the route has great views of the city or the surrounding area. Be sure to bring your camera.

🍴 Somewhere along the route you will have the chance to get food or a beverage. You will have to glance through the walk description to determine where and what kind of food and beverages are available. Walks without the food icon probably are set along nature trails or in noncommercial areas of the city.

🛒 During your walk you will have the chance to shop. More-detailed descriptions of the types of stores you will find can be found in the actual walk description.

👫 This walk has something kids will enjoy seeing or doing—a park, zoo, museum, or play equipment. In most cases the walks that feature this icon are shorter and follow an easy, fairly level path. You know your young walking companions best; if your children are patient walkers who do not tire easily, then feel free to choose walks that are longer and harder. In fact, depending on a child's age and energy, most children can do any of the walks in this book. The icon only notes those walks that are especially good for children.

🏢 Your path will take you primarily through urban areas. Buildings, small city parks, and paved paths are what you will see and pass.

🍃 You will pass through a large park or walk in a natural setting where you can see and enjoy nature.

♿ This icon means that the path is fully accessible and is an easy walk for anyone pushing a wheelchair or stroller. We have made every attempt to follow a high standard for accessibility. The icon means there are curb cuts or ramps along the entire route, plus a wheelchair-accessible bathroom somewhere along the course. The path is mostly or entirely paved, and ramps and nonpaved surfaces are clearly described. If you use a wheelchair and have the ability to negotiate curbs and dirt paths, or to wheel for longer distances and on uneven surfaces, you may want to skim the directions for the walks that do not carry this symbol. You may find other walks you will enjoy. If in doubt, read the full text of the walk or call the contact source for guidance.

(A note to joggers: Joggers also can enjoy many of the walks in this book. If you prefer to jog, first look for those walks with an easy rating. These walks most likely are flat and have a paved or smooth surface. If you want something more challenging, read the walk descriptions to see if the harder routes also appeal to you.)

At the start of each walk chapter, you will find more detailed and specific information that describes the route and what you can expect on your walk:

General location: Here you will get the walk's general location in the city or within a specific area.

Special attractions: Look here to find the specific things you will pass. If this walk has museums, historic homes, restaurants, or wildlife, it will be noted here.

Difficulty: We have designed or selected walking routes that an ordinary person in reasonable health can complete. The walks are rated easy, moderate, or difficult. The ease or difficulty does not relate to a person's level of physical fitness. A walk rated as *Easy* can be completed by an average walker, but that walker may feel tired when he or she has completed the walk and may feel some muscle soreness.

How easy or hard something is depends on each person. But here are some general guidelines of what the ratings mean:

A walk rated as *Easy* is flat, with few or no hills. Most likely you will be walking on a maintained surface made of concrete, asphalt, wood, or packed dirt. The path will be easy to follow, and you will be only a block or so from a phone, other people, or businesses. If the walk is less than a mile, you may be able to walk comfortably in street shoes.

A walk rated as *Moderate* includes some hills, and a few may be steep. The path may include stretches of sand, dirt, gravel, or small crushed rock. The path is easy to follow, but you may not always have street or sidewalk signs, so you may have to check your map or directions. You may be as much as a half-mile from the nearest business or people. You should wear walking shoes.

A walk rated as *Difficult* probably has an unpaved path that includes rocks and patches of vegetation. The trail may have steep ups and downs, and you may have to pause now and then to interpret the walk directions against the natural setting. You will have to carry water, and you may be alone for long stretches during the walk. Walking shoes are a must, and hiking boots may be helpful.

Distance: This gives the total distance of the walk in miles.

Estimated time: The time allotted for each walk is based on walking time only, which is calculated at about 30 minutes per mile—a slow pace. Most people have no trouble walking 1 mile in 30 minutes, and people with some walking experience often walk a 20-minute mile. If the walk includes museums, shops, or restaurants, add sightseeing time to the estimate.

Services: Here you will find out if such things as restrooms, parking, refreshments, or information centers are available, and where you are likely to find them.

Restrictions: The most often noted restriction is pets, which almost always have to be leashed in a city. Most cities also have strict "pooper-scooper" laws, and they enforce them. But restrictions may also include the hours or days a museum or business is open, age requirements, or whether you can ride a bike on the path. If there is something you cannot do on this walk, it will be noted here.

For more information: Each walk includes at least one contact source for you to call for more information. If an agency or business is named as a contact, you will find its phone number and address in Appendix B. This appendix also includes contact information for any business or agency mentioned anywhere in the book.

Getting started: Here you will find specific directions to the starting point. All of these walks are closed loops, which means they begin and end at the same point. Thus, you do not have to worry about finding your car or your way back to the bus stop when your walk is over.

Some downtown walks can be started at any one of several hotels the walk passes. The directions will be for the main starting point, but this section will tell you if it is possible to pick up the walk at other locations. If you are staying at a downtown hotel, it is likely that a walk passes in front of or near your hotel's entrance.

Public transportation: If it is possible to take a bus, streetcar, or MAX train to the walk's starting point, you will find that noted here.

Overview: Every part of a city has a story. Here is where you will find the story or stories about the people, neighborhoods, and history connected to your walk.

The Walk: When you reach this point, you are ready to start walking. In this section you will find specific and detailed directions, and you will also learn more about the things you pass. Those who want only the directions and none of the extras can find the straightforward directions by looking for the arrow symbol.

What to Wear

The best advice is to wear something comfortable. Leave behind anything that binds, pinches, rides up, falls down, slips off the shoulder, or comes undone. Otherwise, let common sense, the weather, and your own body tell you what to wear.

Your feet take the hardest pounding when you walk, so wear good shoes. Sandals, shoes with noticeable heels, or any shoes you rarely wear are not good choices. Some running shoes make superb walking shoes. Choose running shoes with wide heels, little to no narrowing under the arch, noticeable tread designs, and firm insoles.

If you will be walking in the sun, in the heat of the day, in the wind, or along a route with little to no shade, be sure to take along a hat or scarf. Gloves are a must to keep your hands from chapping in the winter, and sunscreen is important year-round.

What to Take

Be sure to take water. Strap a bottle to your pack or tuck a small bottle in a pocket. If you are walking several miles with a dog, remember to take a small bowl so that your pet can also have a drink.

Carry some water even if you will be walking where refreshments are available. Several small sips taken throughout a walk are more effective than one large drink at the walk's end. Also avoid drinks with caffeine or alcohol because they deplete rather than replenish your body's fluids.

If you will be gone for several hours and will walk where there are few or no services, a light backpack can carry beverages, snacks, and other small items.

Safety and Street Savvy

Mention a big city and many people immediately think of safety. Some common questions are: "Is it safe to walk during the day—and what about at night?" and "What areas should I avoid?"

Safety should be a commonsense concern whether you are walking in a small town or a big city, but it does not have to be your overriding concern. America's cities are enjoyable places, and if you follow some basic tips, you will find that these cities are also safe places.

Any safety mishap in a large city is likely to come from petty theft and vandalism, so, the most important tip is a simple one: Do not tempt thieves. Purses dangling on shoulder straps or slung over your arm, wallets peeking out of pockets, arms burdened with packages, valuables on the car seat—all of these things attract the pickpocket, purse snatcher, or thief because you look like someone who could easily be relieved of your possessions.

Do not carry a purse. Put your money in a money belt, or tuck your wallet in a deep side pocket of your pants or skirt. Lock your valuables in the trunk of your car before you park and leave for your walk. Protect your camera by wearing the strap across your chest, not just over your shoulder. Better yet, put your camera in a backpack.

You also will feel safer if you remember the following:

- Be aware of your surroundings and the people near you.
- Avoid parks or other isolated places at night.
- Walk with others.
- Walk in well-lit and well-traveled areas.
- Stop and ask directions if you get lost.

Portland has good cellphone service, though signals sometimes disappear in occasional spots. Usually a little more walking will get you within range. However, make sure your devices are fully charged before you leave on a walk.

The walks in this book were selected by people who had safety in mind. No walk will take you through a bad neighborhood, or into an area known to be dangerous. Relax, pay attention, and enjoy your walk.

Walk Name	Difficulty	Miles	Time	📷	🍴	🛍	👪	🏢	🍂	♿
1. Riverfront and Old Town	Easy	3	2	X	X	X	X	X		X
2. Civic Center/Urban Renewal	Easy	3.25	2	X	X	X	X	X		X
3. The Cultural District	Easy	3.25	1.5	X	X	X	X	X		X
4. The Pearl and Chinatown	Easy	3	2		X	X	X	X		X
5. Northwest Alphabet District	Mod	4	2.5	X	X	X		X		
6. Goose Hollow, Kings Hill and the West End	Mod	3	1.5	X	X	X		X		
7. Audubon Bird Sanctuary	Mod	1	1	X					X	
8. Washington Park North	Mod	2	1	X				X	X	
9. Washington Park South	Easy	2.5	2	X			X	X	X	X
10. Hoyt Arboretum Evergreen Trail	Mod	2	1.5	X					X	
11. Hoyt Arboretum Bristlecone Trail	Easy	.5	½ Hr.	X					X	X

Walk									
12. South Portland—Lair Hill Neighborhood	Mod	3	1.5	X			X		
13. South Portland—Corbett Neighborhood	Mod	3	1.5	X			X		
14. Willamette Greenway	Easy	3	2	X		X			X
15. South Waterfront Parks	Easy	3	2	X		X		X	X
16. Eastbank Esplanade	Easy	3	2				X		X
17. Eastmoreland, Crystal Springs and Reed College	Easy	2.5	1.5	X			X		X
18. Mt. Tabor Park	Mod	2	1			X		X	
19. Convention Center and Lloyd Center	Easy	4	2	X	X	X	X		X
20. Beverly Cleary's Neighborhood*	Easy	7	4	X	X	X	X		X
21. The Grotto	Easy	1	2				X		X
22. East Airport Way	Easy	1.5	½ Hr.	X	X		X		X

*may be divided into two walks

Meet Portland

Fast Facts

General
County: Multnomah. Along with Washington and Clackamas Counties, these make up the tri-county region of the Portland metropolitan area. The surrounding counties of Columbia and Yamhill (Oregon) and Clark (Washington) are also part of the metropolitan area.

Time zone: Pacific. Clocks spring forward on the second Sunday in March, and fall back on the first Sunday of November.

Area code: 503

Size
Oregon's largest city
582,130 people
1.4 million people in metro area
130 square miles

Geographic location
Elevation: 173 feet above sea level
Latitude: 40 miles east of the west 122nd meridian
Longitude: 30 miles north of the 45th parallel (halfway mark between the North Pole and the equator)
Miles to the Pacific Ocean: 78
Miles to Mount Hood: 65

Climate
Average yearly precipitation: 36 inches
Average yearly days of sunshine: 66

Average yearly snowfall: Seldom more than a couple of inches per year

Maximum average temperature: 80 degrees F (may get higher on summer days)

Minimum average temperature: 38.5 degrees F (may get colder during cold snaps)

Average humidity: 60 percent

Average temperatures: 46 degrees F in January; 79.5 degrees F in July

Getting there

Major highways:

Interstates: I-5, I-84, I-205, I-405

US highways: US 30, US 26

State highways: 99E

Airport service: Most domestic airlines and some international airlines, including Air Canada, Alaska, American, Delta, Frontier, Hawaiian, Horizon Air, JetBlue, Seaport, Southwest, Spirit, United, USAirways, and Virgin.

Rail: Amtrak comes into Union Station.

TriMet is the public transit system operating the bus and MAX light-rail lines. The Portland Streetcar connects with the MAX and buses at Pioneer Square. There is also a seasonal, privately run Hop-on Hop-off Trolley going through the downtown area. These all have fees. Call (503) 238-RIDE between 7:30 a.m. and 5:30 p.m. during the week for current times and fares, or check the online Trip Planner service (trimet.org).

Bridges: Ten bridges link Portland's east and west sides by carrying pedestrian and auto traffic over the Willamette River. The oldest of these is the Hawthorne Bridge, built in 1910, and the oldest lift bridge in the world. A new pedestrian and light rail bridge between the Markham and the Ross Island Bridges is scheduled to open in 2015. The Sellwood Bridge will remain open during its remodeling.

Recreation

Golf courses: 13 within city limits; 10 are public. The web page golflink.com/golf-courses gives full information on these.

Parks: There are 37,000 acres in more than 200 parks in the metro area.

Boat tours: The Portland Spirit Company has five ships, three of which begin their cruises at the Salmon Street Park. See their website portlandspirit, or phone (800) 224-3901 for full and current information about their various ships and cruises.

Major industries

Commercial trade, electronics, machinery, food products, transportation equipment.

Media

Television stations:

ABC—Channel 2

CBS—Channel 6

NBC—Channel 8

PBS—Channel 10

Fox—Channel 12

Radio stations:

KXL 750 AM—All news and weather

KOPB 91.5 FM—Oregon Public Broadcasting

Newspapers:

The Oregonian, morning daily

Willamette Week, free weekly tabloid, covers movies, nightclubs, music, art, books, drama, other events

Portland Tribune, free weekly covering local news

Special annual events

Call (800) 962-3700 for a visitor's guide, or use the website (pova.com). Call the Rose Quarter Event Hotline at (503) 321-3211 for events at the Rose Garden or Memorial Coliseum.

April—Tryon Creek State Park Trillium Festival

June—Portland Rose Festival (a month of events)

July—Oregon Brewers Festival

July—Waterfront Blues Festival

July—Multnomah County Fair

August—The Bite: A Taste of Portland

October—Portland Marathon

October—Annual Greek Festival

October—Wordstock Festival (Literary)

December—Christmas Ships: Parade of Lights

December—Zoolights Festival

Weather

Portland enjoys a mild climate year-round. July is the warmest month, with an average temperature of 80 degrees F. January is the coldest, with an average temperature of 36.2 degrees F. Few days have measurable snow.

Despite the jokes, annual rainfall is less than that found in many other major cities. (It just falls more often between October and May.) An entire day of rainfall may measure less than a quarter-inch, so you can generally walk year-round.

Summer days are usually sunny, with low humidity. However, nights are generally cool, so bring along a sweater or jacket. Dressing in layers is a good idea year-round.

Getting Around

For the latest information, check the website travelport land.com/transportation.

I-5 runs north and south through the city, and I-84 brings in traffic from the east. Most addresses are easy to find, since most avenues are numbered, beginning at the Willamette River. The numbering runs to the west on the west side of the river, and to the east on the east side. The larger the number, the farther away you are from downtown.

Portland is divided into five areas: Northeast, Southeast, Northwest, Southwest, and North. Burnside Street divides the north and south parts of the city, while the Willamette River divides east from west. The north side of the city is north of I-405 and mostly west of I-5. House numbers begin at zero from Burnside, with numbers increasing to the north and to the south.

In Portland, you'll find an award-winning airport, efficient light rail system, pedestrian-friendly city blocks, and miles and miles of bike paths—all of which make getting around town a real pleasure.

By air: Portland International Airport is on the northeast side of the city along the Columbia River. Buses and the MAX light rail bring you downtown in less than half an hour.

Zipcar rentals are available throughout Portland's downtown. Phone (503) 328-3539 or check zipcar.com

Safety

The Association for Portland Progress and the City of Portland created the Downtown Clean & Safe Services District to make sure the downtown was a safe, inviting, and lively place for businesses, residents, and visitors. Operation of the district is paid for with a business license fee paid by property managers and building owners, and provides security, crime prevention, and cleaning services in the 212-block downtown area.

The Portland Guides are one of these innovative services. These guides in kelly-green jackets and caps roam the downtown seven days a week in teams of two. They are trained to offer assistance, answer questions, and make sure visitors feel welcome. Police officers also continually patrol downtown.

Fair-weather evenings and special events always bring people out, and the well-lit areas that are busy with people are generally safe for walkers. Otherwise, as in most cities, it is best to walk during daylight hours.

The Story of Portland

When emigrants on the Oregon Trail reached a fork in the trail, one story says, they had to make a decision about which way to go. One trail was marked with a lump of gold ore. The other had a sign reading TO OREGON. Those who wanted riches went to California, while those who could read came to Oregon. Despite the implications of this apocryphal story, Oregon also attracted entrepreneurs who hoped to make money.

After Lewis and Clark returned from their famous expedition with glowing news of the lands they had discovered, the United States needed an answer to the British settlement at Fort Vancouver. Oregon City, a town at the falls farther up the Willamette River, was founded in 1829 as the first major settlement in Oregon. Francis W. Pettygrove, an employee of a New York City merchant, was sent to Oregon City to open a store. Asa Lovejoy, who originally visited Oregon with missionary Marcus Whitman, saw the town as an ideal place to practice law.

The Clearing

William Overton, the first man to file a land claim on the site that became Portland, was a drifter who was searching for golden opportunities. He staked a claim on a popular camping spot for sailors and traders. It was known as "The Clearing" because over the years the trees had been cut down to feed campfires. Overton offered a half interest in his claim to Lovejoy in return for Lovejoy's filing the claim and paying the 25-cent filing fee. Overton soon decided to move on, and he traded the other half of his claim to Pettygrove in return for $50 worth of supplies.

Another man who was impressed by this clearing was Massachusetts sea captain John H. Couch (pronounced "kooch"), one of the first to bring a ship filled with merchandise up the Willamette River to Oregon City. However, on a subsequent trip, he was unable to navigate that far, and he realized that the site of the Lovejoy-Pettygrove claim would make a better port. He then took up a land claim to the north.

Couch, Lovejoy, and Pettygrove were all profit-seeking entrepreneurs. They were also educated men who brought their knowledge of the world to the frontier. Pettygrove, from Maine, had lived in New York City. Lovejoy was educated at colleges in Amherst and Cambridge, Massachusetts, and had visited many of the great cities of the world. The ideas they had about what constituted a proper city helped to give Portland a good start.

Lovejoy and Pettygrove hired surveyor Thomas Brown to lay out "The Clearing" in a 16-block grid of 200-square-foot blocks and 60-foot-wide streets. They numbered the north-south avenues, starting at the Willamette. They gave names to the east-west streets. They also dedicated some of the blocks for public use. Pettygrove built a wharf at the foot of what is now Washington Street, and began a road up to the farming area known as the Tualatin Plains. At this point, both men thought the town needed a more dignified name. Lovejoy proposed "Boston," while Pettygrove preferred "Portland." The choice was settled with the toss of a copper coin.

Stumptown

Portland has always had a number of affectionate and not-so-affectionate nicknames that reflect the city's development. Even after the town acquired its first official name, it was usually called "Stumptown" because of the numerous stumps left standing in the streets as trees were cut down to supply building materials. Even when white-washed, the stumps were a traffic hazard.

In 1848, as the town began to prosper, Lovejoy and Pettygrove sold their claims to Daniel Lownsdale and merchant Benjamin Stark. Lawyer William Chapman and builder Stephen Coffin also purchased land in what is now the downtown area. They began clearing the stumps from the streets, and Lownsdale started another road to the Tualatin Valley. Chapman, who had previously tried to start a railroad, joined Coffin in constructing this plank road so that farmers could bring their produce to town more easily.

By 1859, when Oregon became a state, more than 200 buildings filled the Portland streets. Together, Lownsdale, Chapman, Coffin, Stark, and Couch dedicated more land to public use, including 25 blocks for a park boulevard through the center of the city. These blocks, now known as the Park Blocks, are one of Portland's best-loved features.

The River City

By this time, the town was a thriving port. As the Civil War heated up, emigrants from both sides of the controversy poured into Oregon via the Oregon Trail.

Prospectors came and went, leaving the merchants to make good money. The heavy river commerce attracted longshoremen and Chinese dockworkers. Vicious rivalry and competition developed among the steamship companies, until the Oregon Steam Navigation Company monopolized traffic on both the Columbia and Willamette. Later, some rival companies sprang up, and the railroad was finally completed. The town became known for some of its notorious citizens, such as Joseph Kelly, who bragged that he could shanghai a full crew of men for any ship in less than twelve hours. "Sweet Mary" was the madam of a floating bordello that ran up and down the river, avoiding both the law and taxes.

The White City

By the late 1800s, the town had stabilized. The "Great Fire" of 1873 had destroyed all the wooden buildings in twenty-two downtown blocks, but they had been replaced with more-permanent structures, often with cast-iron facades. The completed railroad brought visitors to the city, and a fine hotel became necessary. Railroader Henry Villard hired famous Eastern architect Stanford White to design what became the well-loved Portland Hotel. White's assistant, A. E. Doyle, had been fascinated by the "City Beautiful" ideas displayed at the 1893 World's Fair and Columbian Exposition in Chicago, and he hoped to make Portland a "White City" using terra-cotta trim. Doyle was soon hired by many prospering merchants to implement his ideas, and many of Doyle's buildings still survive today.

Seattle had hired the famous Olmsted Brothers landscape firm to develop their park system. John C. Olmsted, son of the firm's founder, Frederick Olmsted, was sent to the Northwest. While here, he was hired to make suggestions for additions and improvements to Portland's city park system. Many of his ideas have slowly been adopted through the years.

The Bridge City

As the city grew on both sides of the Willamette, bridges were needed to connect the two areas. The first bridge was built in 1887, and others soon followed. Today, ten bridges connect the two sides of the Willamette. Five of these open to allow the passage of river traffic; the others are fixed.

The city east of the river has continued to grow and has conveniently continued the system of numbering all north-south streets. No matter where you are in Portland, it's easy to find your way around.

The City of Roses

The Lewis and Clark Centennial Exposition of 1905 brought a great deal of positive attention to Portland, and civic leaders wished to capitalize on the publicity. Since roses were thriving in Portland's gardens—Georgiana Pittock staged the first rose show at her home in 1888—Mayor Harry Lane proposed a Festival of Roses to begin in 1907. The International Rose Test Gardens were installed in Washington Park in 1917, and roses have been synonymous with Portland ever since.

The City that Works

This somewhat boastful motto, seen on many municipal vehicles, has some truth to it. Portland has preserved and built on the best of its past. The vision and civic generosity of Portland's founders have enhanced today's city life. Lovejoy's small "dollhouse blocks" make the city a pedestrian's delight. Doyle's "white" buildings light up the downtown.

Today's civic leaders have vision, too. Most older public buildings are surrounded by lawns and fill an entire block.

The city code requires newer buildings to include shops and courtyards at sidewalk level. The Metropolitan Art for Public Places Act, enacted in 1980, requires that 1 percent of all municipal building costs be allocated to on-site art, and many privately funded buildings have followed suit, so an eclectic assortment of art pieces delights passersby.

The Outdoor City

Today, the "Outdoor City" might be an appropriate nickname for Portland. Its green spaces and sanctuaries didn't just happen. In 1904, the Olmsted brothers visualized a 40-mile loop of parks and boulevards surrounding the city. This vision is slowly being realized in what is still called the "40-Mile Loop," although when completed it will be a 130-mile trail connecting municipal parks with others along the Willamette, Columbia, and Sandy Rivers. Tom McCall Waterfront Park, created by tearing down an expressway, was backed by and named for the former visionary and governor.

The Ever-Changing City

As I have re-walked Portland this past year, I have certainly noticed how Portland has changed in both big and small ways. This is probably true of many cities, but it seems especially true of Portland these past years. Downtown art pieces and fountains have been moved, a new floating bridge has been built for pedestrians and bicyclists, and more major, walk-friendly public works are on the way. New parks have been added in various parts of the city. My area of the city, barely mentioned in 1998, is now a growing, user-friendly, and ecologically sustainable neighborhood. Public transportation is reaching more neighborhoods, although the free zones are gone. Many chafe at zoning rules and regulations, but the end results seem to have made the city more livable as well as more walkable. What began as a simple revision of a walk or two has evolved into an almost completely new book. The city truly is ever-changing.

One thing will never change, and that is Portland's beautiful setting between mountains, rivers, and ocean. The welcome mat is still out. Come and mingle with those who have come to love this city. As you walk, enjoy your surroundings, and choose your own nickname for this lovely corner of the Pacific Northwest.

DOWNTOWN

Walk 1: Riverfront and Old Town

📷 ✕ 🛒 👫 🏢 ♿

General location: Downtown Portland, west of I-5

Special attractions: Historic buildings, interesting shops and restaurants, and the Willamette River waterfront

Difficulty: Easy, flat; entirely on paved sidewalks with curb cuts

Distance: 3 miles

Estimated time: 2 hours

Services: Restaurants, restrooms, tourist information center

Restrictions: Days and hours vary at the museums. Check with the Visitor Center for current information. The 2012 hours at the Nikkei Legacy Center are 11 a.m. to 3 p.m., Tuesday through Saturday, and Sunday from noon to 3 p.m. The Maritime Museum is open Wednesday, Friday, Saturday, and Sunday from 12:30 to 4:30 p.m.

For more information: Portland Tourist Information can be found at travelportland.com or at the visitor center in Pioneer Square. 701 Southwest 6th Avenue, Portland, OR 97204; (503) 275-8355.

Getting started: The walk begins at the World Trade Center Conference Center, Building 2, between Salmon & Taylor, on Naito Parkway. (Naito was formerly named Front Avenue, which is still shown on older maps.)

Public transportation: The World Trade Center is half a mile from the MAX station at Morrison and 1st Avenue.

Overview: This riverfront area is where Portland was originally founded and developed. Fires destroyed the early wooden buildings, which were replaced by buildings with cast-iron facades. After major downtown flooding in the late 1800s, businesses moved back from the river, leaving these buildings behind. Many old structures were demolished. Those remaining are now being renovated, restored, and reused by enticing shops and restaurants.

An expressway along the riverbank was torn down to create Tom McCall Waterfront Park. Today this entrance to the city hosts many civic and cultural events. It is always full of walkers, cyclers, runners, dogs, and people just admiring the view.

The Walk

▶Begin at the World Trade Center, Building 2, on the northwest corner of Salmon Street and Naito Parkway, opposite the Salmon Street Fountain. Inside the lobby of this building is a miniature version of *Portlandia,* Portland's iconic statue. The original *Portlandia* sculpture peers down at passersby from the second-floor front of the Portland Building on 5th Avenue and Main Street, but this gives you an up-close and personal chance to appraise her features.

▶Exit, and go north on Naito to Taylor Street. Cross Taylor. A plaque at this corner tells about tiny Mill Ends Park, located in the Naito Parkway traffic island. Dick Fagan, a newspaper columnist, grew tired of seeing an empty hole beneath his office window. He filled it with flowers, dedicated it on

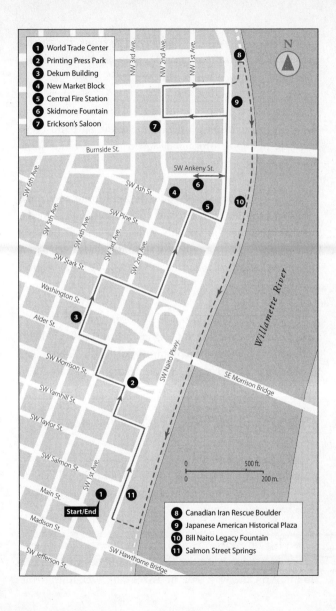

1 World Trade Center
2 Printing Press Park
3 Dekum Building
4 New Market Block
5 Central Fire Station
6 Skidmore Fountain
7 Erickson's Saloon

8 Canadian Iran Rescue Boulder
9 Japanese American Historical Plaza
10 Bill Naito Legacy Fountain
11 Salmon Street Springs

NW 3rd Ave.
NW 2nd Ave.
NW 1st Ave.

Burnside St.

SW Ankeny St.

SW 6th Ave.
SW 5th Ave.
SW 4th Ave.
SW 3rd Ave.
SW 2nd Ave.
SW 1st Ave.

SW Ash St.
SW Pine St.
SW Stark St.
Washington St.
Alder St.
SW Morrison St.
SW Yamhill St.
SW Taylor St.
SW Salmon St.
Main St.
Madison St.
SW Jefferson St.

SW Naito Pkwy.

SE Morrison Bridge

Willamette River

SW Hawthorne Bridge

Start/End

N

0   500 ft.
0   200 m.

St. Patrick's Day, 1948, as "the only leprechaun colony west of Ireland," and wrote occasional columns about the leprechauns. It was given official status in 1976.

▶Cross to the traffic island to see the world's smallest park. Across Naito on the park side is one of the Portland Loos, hygienic public bathrooms designed to serve basic needs and discourage other uses.

▶Stay on the west side of Naito and continue north one block to Yamhill. Turn left and go to 1st Avenue. On the northwest corner of 1st and Yamhill is the Willamette Block Building, one example of the old Italianate cast-iron buildings for which this district is noted. A MAX station is in front of it.

▶Turn right and then go north on the east side of 1st Avenue. Cross Morrison into Oregonian Printing Press Park, another small park commemorating Portland's oldest major newspaper, still publishing. Six display signs bear reproductions of front pages announcing significant world events.

▶Turn left, cross 1st, and go west to 2nd Avenue.

▶Turn right on 2nd and continue to Alder Street. As you walk, look left. The entrance to the Oregon Dental Service Tower here is surrounded by a giant cedar tree, enhanced with twining metal vines.

▶Turn left on Alder Street to 3rd Avenue. Turn right and go one block north. Notice the Romanesque-style Dekum Building on the west side of 3rd. Frank Dekum left the

California goldfields with only $2 in his pocket, but made a Portland fortune in merchandising and banking. Only local materials were used for this substantial-looking building. A king's head and carved griffins adorn the massive doorway arch, and the lower three stories are faced with sandstone. The upper redbrick stories are decorated with terra-cotta garlands.

▶Cross Washington, passing the food carts on the east side of 3rd. Note Portland's oldest restaurant, Huber's, founded twenty years after Oregon became a state. It has been at this present site since 1910 and is still run by the same family, whose Chinese ancestor was first hired as a turkey slicer for sandwiches. During a flood he kept working, slicing turkey from a rowboat behind the bar. The mahogany panels and stained-glass skylights are original, crafted by the Povey Brothers who created most of Portland's stained glass windows. They give you the feeling of being back in the early twentieth century.

▶Turn right on Stark Street, and proceed toward 2nd Avenue. At mid-block note the slender Gothic-style Bishop's House across Stark. This building, originally constructed in 1879 as an addition to a Roman Catholic cathedral that once stood next door, was restored in 1965. Cross 2nd and proceed to 1st Avenue.

▶Turn left (north) at 1st, crossing Stark, and then proceed to Oak Street. You have entered the Skidmore / Old Town Historic District. The building on your left at the northwest corner of 1st and Oak is the 1886 Failing Building, built in a French and Italian style of architecture. Looking east on Oak toward the river at 71 SW Oak is the 1859 Dielschneider Building, the third-oldest commercial brick building in Portland. Note the ironwork facade.

▸Cross Oak and go one block north on 1st. Cross Pine, noticing the varied architectural styles on the east side of the street.

▸Cross Ash with the traffic signal. Turn right toward the river, passing the New Market Block with its classic cast-iron features at the northwest corner.

▸Continue to the Central Fire Station. Note the beautiful stained-glass windows (featuring fire engines) around the front door. Enter the vestibule to see the large 1911 American LaFrance horse-drawn steamer adorned with paint and gold-leaf trim by Mitch Kim. This is thought to be one of the finest in the world. The engine, restored by Portland fire-fighters Al Carocci and Frank Maas, is pulled by firefighters each June in the annual Rose Festival Starlight Parade.

▸Exit the vestibule and look toward the river. In the 1880s the steamship docks were at this end of Ash.

▸Turn left on Naito Parkway, passing by the window that gives another view of this engine. Pass the station and turn left at Ankeny Square to 1st Avenue. Note a variety of cast-iron ornaments on this north wall of the station. Turn left on 1st Avenue to read the "Ankeny Arcade" sign, which describes how these buildings were salvaged when the original ones were torn down. Return to the elegant

Skidmore Fountain, with basins of water for "horses, men, and dogs." On the west side of 1st Avenue is the New Market Theater, which once had a drive-through market.

SKIDMORE FOUNTAIN

Stephen Skidmore, founder of a major "pharmaceutical emporium," was a prominent member of Portland society in 1870. Fountains he saw during a European tour impressed him so much that he left a bequest for one of this type to be built here in Portland. He stipulated that it provide water "for horses, men, and dogs."

Colonel Charles Erskine Wood—soldier, lawyer, poet, artist, and lifelong friend of the famous Nez Perce Chief Joseph—knew many people associated with the Eastern art establishment. Appointed to carry out Skidmore's bequest, he chose famous New York sculptor Olin Warner. Warner's wife supposedly modeled for one of the supporting bronze caryatids. Wood added the motto, "Good citizens are the riches of a city."

The fountain was shipped from New York City by rail and installed in this central location in 1888. Some Portland citizens—and even a New York newspaper—complained that the creation was too artistic for upstart Portland. Then nearby brewer Henry Weinhard offered to pipe in a "beer of the day." Can you imagine what the critics would have said if this offer had been accepted?

▸The Packer-Scott Building forms the north side of the square. Originally a warehouse, it now serves as the international headquarters for Mercy Corps. One of the two arched colonnades here came from Captain Ankeny's 1883 brick building on this site. The Portland Friends of Cast-Iron Architecture saved the other colonnade from another demolished building. The arches make marvelous frames for photographs.

▸Walk east through the colonnades to Naito Parkway. The Lewis and Clark Memorial sign at the corner of Ankeny informs you that some botanical specimens brought back by this expedition are planted in the waterfront park across the street.

▸Ankeny is the first of the streets laid on a true north grid, rather than the earlier plan oriented with the river. From here the east-west streets are in alphabetical order.

▸Cross Ankeny, continue north, and go under the Burnside Bridge. Burnside is the dividing line between Portland's north- and south-side districts. From here on going north, the street signs will be labeled NW. This area of Old Town contains a diverse mixture of artists, crafters, seniors, businesspeople, and those living on the street for a variety of reasons. The sight of some of the "street people" makes some tourists uncomfortable, but the local merchants work hard to keep the area free from trouble, and the district is considered safe for tourists.

The long-running Saturday (and Sunday) craft market began here under the bridge. It is open from mid-March through Christmas Eve. Craft and food vendors offer unique handmade items in this, the largest open-air craft market in the country. All crafts are juried to meet the market's high standards.

▶Pass the Skidmore Building with the neon white stag sign on the roof. Continue north to Couch Street, past the Blagen Block Building—the last remaining Italianate "commercial palace."

This particular area was part of the land claim of John Couch, the veteran seaman from Newburyport, Massachusetts, who thought this was the best site for a port. When he acquired his extensive land claim running west to 23rd Avenue, he laid it out on true north, so he could see the North Star he had sailed by at the end of his platted streets. He also named them with the letters of the alphabet. In later years, the letters were replaced by names of early Portland leaders, still in alphabetical order.

▶Turn left on Couch, crossing 1st Avenue to the Norton House, a former hotel where President Ulysses S. Grant stayed briefly.

▶Continue west to 2nd Avenue. You are now opposite the 1906 Fleischner-Mayer Building, once a dry-goods store. This was one of the first buildings restored by the Naito brothers, members of the Japanese-American family that began this area's rejuvenation.

▶Cross 2nd. The sign located mid-block on the building on your left provides information about the history of Erickson's Saloon. Loggers and sailors once frequented its 672-foot-long bar. Supposedly, many drunken unfortunates

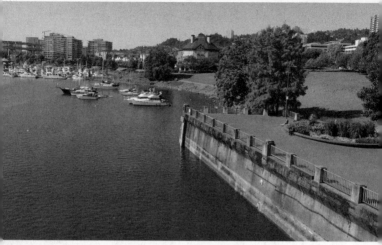

Enjoy a lovely waterfront view along the promenade.

were dropped through a trapdoor to the tunnels beneath the streets. The second floor was reserved for higher society, so they could look down on the riffraff.

▸Turn right on 2nd, crossing Couch, and walk north toward Davis. The Nikkei Legacy Center on your left has many exhibits and archives relating to this period, including a model of what was once considered "Japantown." The museum is part of the Merchant Hotel, an important center for immigrants.

▸Turn left on Davis. A small alley on your left goes into the original courtyard of the hotel, still used for rentals. The windows of the Old Town Pizza Restaurant are on your left. The restaurant is the starting point for Portland

Underground Tours, which offers you the chance to visit the tunnels where the shanghaied sailors ended up.

▶Return to and cross 2nd Avenue. Go two blocks to Naito Parkway, formerly known as Front Avenue. Front was the first paved street in Portland.

▶Use the push button for the walk signal on the street post, then cross Naito Parkway into Tom McCall Waterfront Park.

▶Turn left on the sidewalk, taking the steps down to the river promenade, and look for the boulder on the left; it features a brass plaque honoring the Canadian embassy in

ON JANUARY 28, 1980, CANADIAN EMISSARIES IN IRAN RISKED THEIR LIVES BY SHELTERING SIX AMERICANS WHO WERE OUTSIDE OF THE AMERICAN EMBASSY DURING THE TIME OF ITS SEIZURE. WE, THE PEOPLE OF THE CITY OF PORTLAND, HONOR CANADA FOR OFFERING SANCTUARY TO THE AMERICANS. CANADA'S NOBLE ACT IN BRINGING THE AMERICANS HOME CALLS FORTH OUR PROFOUND GRATITUDE AND APPRECIATION.

This plaque thanks Canada for rescuing American embassy workers from Iran (1980).

Iran. After the 1979 Islamic Revolution, Muslim students imprisoned American Embassy workers for 444 days. Several diplomats who managed to flee the embassy were eventually hidden in the Canadian embassy, at great risk to the Canadian ambassador. This is a thank-you for what became known as the "Canadian Caper."

▶The green glass towers on the other side of the river belong to the Oregon Convention Center. Turn south on the walkway until you come to a stone path leading to the right. Take this into the Japanese-American Historical Plaza, a reminder of the days when American citizens were forced to leave their homes for relocation camps. It is highlighted by two bronze cylinders, *Songs of Innocence* and *Songs of Experience,* carved with sketches of soldiers and civilians. It is sometimes referred to as the "stone garden" for its use of stones. The fractured pavement in the center of the plaza represents the internees' broken dreams.

Thirteen basalt and granite pillars are engraved with verses by Oregon poets in both Japanese and English. The last stone includes a reminder of how the forced internment of Japanese Americans during World War II violated every single article of the US Constitution and the Bill of Rights. It has excerpts from the Civil Liberties Act of 1988, and the official apology by the US Congress for the unlawful imprisonment of US citizens.

▶Turn right on the river walkway as you leave the Japanese-American Historical Plaza and go under the Burnside Bridge. Enjoy the view of Portland's skyline, but watch for bicyclists, runners, and skateboarders who share this river-walk. Also, be on the lookout for the fat iron mooring posts called "bollards," used to moor visiting ships, including those of the US Navy, which arrive each June for the Rose Festival.

▶Walk by the polished, stainless-steel Sculpture Stage, and enter a square featuring the Bill Naito Legacy Fountain. Many of Portland's outdoor activities and festivals take place here. The wide steps, ideal for sitting on, "remember Bill Naito as a businessman and true citizen, son of this Old Town neighborhood, a tireless champion of the preservation of its history and for the potential of its people."

WILLIAM SUMIO NAITO (1925–1996)

Bill Naito was a native Portlander and the son of Japanese immigrants Hide and Fukieye Naito. When World War II began, Congress passed the Wartime Relocation Act, forcing all Japanese-American citizens living on the West Coast to move to internment camps. Naito's family chose instead to move in with relatives in Salt Lake City.

As soon as Naito was old enough, he joined the US Army, serving as a translator. After the war he earned degrees in economics from Reed College and the University of Chicago before returning to Portland to join his brother Sam in the family import business.

Bill Naito began to buy historic buildings and turn them into commercially successful properties. He converted lower floors of his renovated buildings into small shops, and provided low-income housing for neighborhood residents on the upper levels. Naito was convinced that Portland was a great city with

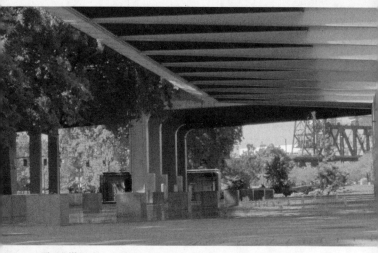

The Bill Naito Legacy Fountain hosts many events and festivals.

an exciting future, and his enthusiasm and creativity are behind many of the buildings seen on these downtown walks. He changed Old Town, donated space for Saturday Market, and began the revival of the downtown core.

►Continue walking south. The ship moored on your left is the *Portland*, the last steam-powered sternwheel tugboat built in the United States, in 1947. Though the tug pilots prized the stern-wheelers for their unique ship-handling ability, diesels finally took over. This ship has been restored by charitable grants and thousands of hours of volunteer work. It doubled as the *Lauren Belle* in the 1994 movie, *Maverick,* and now has a new role as the Oregon Maritime

Museum. It contains many artifacts from Portland's rich seafaring history, and is open to the public. Check the museum website (oregonmaritimemuseum.org) for current schedules. An old navy barge, the *Russell,* is docked in front of the *Portland,* and serves as a workspace for museum volunteers.

▶Look for the smokestack on the far right of the walkway. This is from the battleship USS *Oregon,* which saw action in Cuba during the Spanish-American War. A bicentennial time capsule inside the stack is to be opened in 2076.

▶As you walk along, look down to see markers for sites of early Portland history inscribed in the concrete. Not too far from the *Portland* is one for THE CLEARING, which Captain Couch thought "a good spot for a seaport." Other signs mark "Indian Camps, 1845," the first wharf built in 1846, and a Stephens family's land claim across the river. The next marker designates the 1845 townsite. The Lownsdale land claim marker is at Morrison Street, site of the first bridge built over the Willamette River in 1887.

▶Continue to the Salmon Street Springs fountain. This is a child's delight, with a variety of three spray patterns (bollards, wedding cake, and misters) that seem to change constantly. Steps along the riverside provide a place to sit, admire the river, or wait your turn for a warm-weather river cruise on the *Portland Spirit.*

▶Turn west and cross Naito Parkway at the traffic signal. You have now returned to your starting point at the World Trade Center.

Walk 2: Civic Center / Urban Renewal

■ ✗ 🛒 🏢 ♿

General location: The center of downtown Portland, west of I-5

Special attractions: Government buildings dating from 1869 through 1997, a variety of fountains, old and new parks, a planned integrated area of shops, offices, and apartments

Difficulty: Easy, flat; entirely on paved sidewalk with curb cuts

Distance: 3.25 miles

Estimated time: 2 hours

Services: Restrooms are available at the TriMet offices in Pioneer Courthouse Square and in all public buildings. Most public buildings are open weekdays from 9 a.m. to 5 p.m. Stores and restaurants are located throughout the area. The "Smart Park" city parking garages provide the most inexpensive parking in Portland. There are three in the immediate vicinity. One is on 10th between Yamhill and Morrison, with an entrance on 10th; one is at 3rd Avenue and Alder Street, with entrances on 3rd and 4th; and one is at 4th Avenue and Yamhill, with the entrance on 4th.

Restrictions: The Portland Visitor Information Center is open Monday through Friday, 8:30 a.m. to 5:30 p.m., and Saturday, 10 a.m. to 4 p.m. It is open Sunday from May through October, 10 a.m. to 2 p.m. The TriMet

Transportation Center is open Monday through Friday, 8:30 a.m. to 5:30 p.m., and is closed on national holidays. The Police Museum is open Monday through Thursday, 10 a.m. to 3 p.m.

For more information: Contact the Portland Oregon Visitors Association.

Getting started: This walk begins at Pioneer Courthouse Square, between Broadway and 6th Avenue and Yamhill and Morrison Streets. From I-5 northbound, take the exit to I-405, then take the 6th Avenue exit and continue south to Yamhill Street and Pioneer Courthouse Square. From US 26, take the Market Street exit and follow the City Center signs to 10th Avenue. Turn left on 10th, cross Taylor Street, and turn right on Yamhill for three blocks.

Public transportation: Buses and MAX light-rail lines meet at Pioneer Courthouse Square. The TriMet information station and ticket office is situated below the coffee shop and is open Monday through Friday, 8 a.m. to 5 p.m. Contact TriMet for information about fares and schedules (trimet.org).

Overview: This walk begins at Portland's Pioneer Courthouse Square, center of today's downtown Portland, and easily reached on foot from most downtown hotels. This square has long been the center of the city—first, as the site of the city's first school, and later, the elegant Portland Hotel. The square now serves as a city plaza, transportation hub, and venue for a variety of popular outdoor events. Its backers hoped for the square to be "distinctive, dynamic, elegant, inviting, and unique to the area." Architect Willard Martin's design managed all of that, and the plaza is still a vibrant city center nearly thirty years after its 1984 opening. You will see Portland's oldest

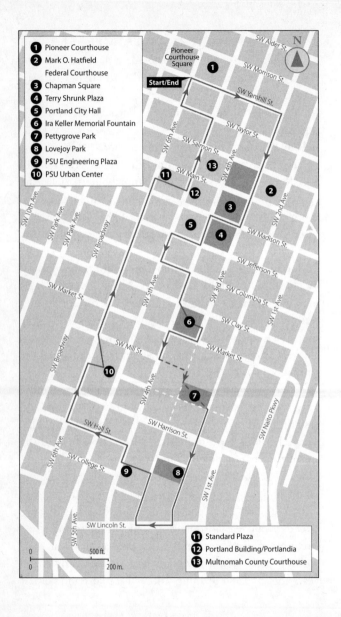

1. Pioneer Courthouse
2. Mark O. Hatfield Federal Courthouse
3. Chapman Square
4. Terry Shrunk Plaza
5. Portland City Hall
6. Ira Keller Memorial Fountain
7. Pettygrove Park
8. Lovejoy Park
9. PSU Engineering Plaza
10. PSU Urban Center

11. Standard Plaza
12. Portland Building/Portlandia
13. Multnomah County Courthouse

SW Alder St.
Pioneer Courthouse Square
SW Morrison St.
Start/End
SW Yamhill St.
SW Taylor St.
SW Salmon St.
SW Main St.
SW 6th Ave
SW 4th Ave
SW 2nd Ave
SW Madison St.
SW Jefferson St.
SW 3rd Ave
SW Columbia St.
SW Clay St.
SW Market St.
SW 10th Ave
SW Park Ave
SW Park Ave
SW Broadway
SW Market St.
SW 5th Ave
SW Mill St.
SW Broadway
SW Hall St.
SW College St.
SW 6th Ave
SW Harrison St.
SW 1st Ave
SW Naito Pkwy
SW 5th Ave
SW Lincoln St.

0   500 ft.
0   200 m.

N

courthouse as well as the newest. The Mark O. Hatfield Federal Courthouse was completed in 1997. The walk continues through Portland Center, an area of integrated housing, shops, and offices often called "New Town," or the "Superblocks."

The Walk

▸Start your walk by the milepost sign on the 6th Avenue side of Pioneer Square. This points outs the direction and mileage to many places in Oregon, and the world, including Portland's nine sister cities: Ashkelon, Israel; Corinto, Nicaragua; Guadalajara, Mexico; Kaosiung Municipality, China; Suzhou, China; Khabarovsk, Russia; Mutare, Zimbabwe; Sapporo, Japan; and Ulsan, Korea.

▸Turn right to Yamhill, then turn left and cross 6th Avenue to the corner of the original Pioneer Courthouse, built in 1869. The small blue structures at this corner once led to underground restrooms. The courthouse, built after the Civil War, was restored in 1873 and again in 2005. Still a working courthouse for the US Court of Appeals, it is open to visitors. Take the stairs or either ramp up to the lobby. Enter to see the large carved wooden figure on the right side of the lobby. The security booth blocks your view of the matching one on the left. Both were carved in Denmark for the former Jacob Kamm Building and were moved here after it was demolished. Go through security to see the other carving, admire the large display of historical photographs, or go up the 115 steps to the cupola for a splendid view of the city.

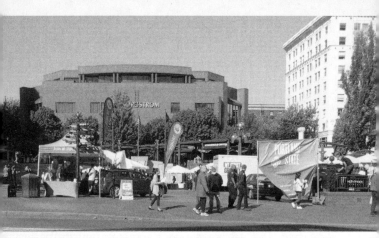

Portland State University exhibit goes up in Portland's central square. *Dick Lukins*

▶Exit the courthouse, return to the corner of 6th and Yamhill, and turn east on Yamhill past the courthouse, to 5th Avenue. Along the sidewalk are Georgia Gerber's frolicsome *Animals in Pools.* Sometimes called "The Bronze Zoo," these sculptures appeal to animal lovers of all ages. The rest of the "zoo" is on the Morrison side of the courthouse.

▶Portland's entire downtown area is home to an interesting collection of outdoor art. In 1975, the state legislature passed a "1 percent for art" program, allocating this amount of state building–construction money for "publicly accessible works of art." Most of these pieces are along the 5th and 6th Avenues transit malls.

▶Cross 5th Avenue. On both sides of Yamhill between 5th and 3rd are the four full blocks of the Pioneer Place Mall.

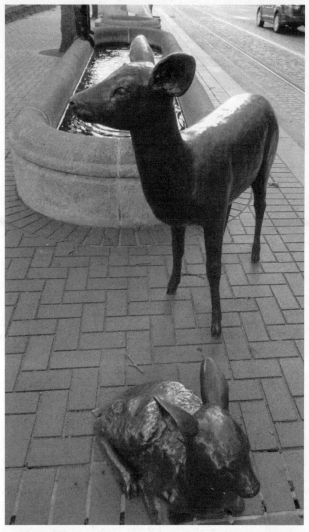

Animals in Pools is one sculpture you'll see in the "Bronze Zoo." *Dick Lukins*

Shops range from the Apple Store to Tiffany's, and include two Oregon specialties: Made in Oregon and Moonstruck Chocolates.

▶Go to 4th Avenue. The blocks on either side are also part of Pioneer Place. Note the plaques enlivening the otherwise blank wall on your right. These explain various city symbols: the gargoyles, the early "Portlandia" silhouette on a city shield, and the rose from which the city takes its nickname.

▶Cross 4th and proceed to 3rd. At your feet and on the wall is *Streetwise,* a work of sidewalk art designed by Portland author Katherine Dunn and artist Bill Will. Quotations from people such as Groucho Marx, Anatole France, Ursula Le Guin, and "Anonymous" are engraved on granite pavement blocks, or on bronze plaques set in the building walls. Expressive terra-cotta faces look down from the upper wall.

▶Turn right on 3rd, go south to Taylor, and cross. Note the redbrick building across the street, mid-block at 920 3rd Avenue. Noted architect Louis Sullivan designed this Auditorium Building. He began the "form follows function" movement, and this is an excellent example of his "Roman column" design. The lower floors make the base, the middle represents the column, and the upper stories are the capitals.

▶Continue to Salmon Street. Cross Salmon to Lownsdale Square. Look across to see the 1997 Mark O. Hatfield Federal Courthouse on the east side. This is the first asymmetrical US courthouse, with different facades on the surrounding streets, making it appear to be three different buildings. If you wish, cross the street and enter the building. You will have to leave your camera or video recorder with the security guards before taking the elevator to the rooftop garden on the ninth floor. The garden has a great view of the city and Willamette River. Enjoy Tom Otterness's delightful and whimsical *Law of Nature,* with small bronze animal figures portraying different aspects of justice. Then return down to Lownsdale Square.

Lownsdale and Chapman Squares, the two Plaza Blocks, were laid out in 1852. These squares were historically "where orators held forth and citizens assembled." Signs in each park give a brief history of the men behind the names. Lownsdale was the "gentlemen's gathering place," and Chapman was meant for women and children. Although both squares have lovely old elms and gingko trees, Chapman's gingkoes are exclusively female. Lownsdale Square is the site of Douglas Tilden's 1906 *Soldiers' Monument,* topped with a soldier of the Second Oregon Volunteer Infantry, part of the first large fighting force ever sent overseas. The small cannons at the base were used at Fort Sumter in the Civil War. One faces north and one faces south, representing their use by both Union and Confederate forces. A drinking fountain on the 4th Avenue side of the park is another memorial to Spanish-American War volunteers.

▸Continue south on 3rd Avenue and cross Main Street. As you cross you can see a large bronze elk on the Main Street traffic island on your right. Drinking troughs for horses and dogs surround the base. Former mayor David Thompson gave this to the city in 1900, and it commemorates a real elk that grazed here regularly in Portland's early days.

Now you are at Chapman Square. Instead of monuments to war, this contains *The Promised Land* sculpture of an idealized pioneer family. Created to celebrate the 150th anniversary of the Oregon Trail, the pavement in front has footprints of moccasin-clad humans and animals found here at that time. See if you can identify the ones made by a jackrabbit, porcupine, black bear, grouse, coyote, and elk.

East across 3rd Avenue is the Justice Center. Travertine pillars flank the entrance, and an arched stained-glass window wall is above the door. The ceiling of the portico is covered with Liz Mapelli's beautiful mosaic of Venetian and fused-glass tiles, and is lit by hanging lamps resembling copper kettledrums. More public art is inside the building. The Portland Police Museum is on the first floor, and admission is free. Contact the museum about hours.

▸Proceed south on 3rd Avenue and cross Madison to the Terry Schrunk Federal Plaza. Its steps and ledges and grassy areas provide pleasant places to perch, and give a good view of the Edith Green–Wendell Wyatt Building, named for two former members of the US House of Representatives. Note the pipe-like bars hanging down in front of the windows, which act as a sunshade.

Schrunk Plaza sits atop the Green/Wyatt Federal Building's parking garage, the site of an attempted 1995 bombing by the Rajneeshees, which targeted the US District Attorney. The Murrah Federal Building in Oklahoma City was bombed in this same year. On the first anniversary of the Oklahoma City bombing, a memorial plaque and piece of the Murrah Building were installed here, on the north side of the top level of the entrance steps. On the south wall is the plaque honoring former mayor Terry Schrunk.

The 16-ton, 22-foot-high Taihu Rock, a gift from Portland's sister city, Suzhou, China, stands out against a large evergreen tree on the west side of the plaza. It comes from the bottom of Lake Tai, where erosion created the interesting surface. (The same type of rock is in Portland's Lan Su Chinese Garden.) The Chinese wanted it near City Hall, and its weight finally mandated its placement atop a large structural column in the parking garage underneath the park.

▸Exit back at 3rd and Madison. Turn west on the plaza's north side to 4th Avenue and cross. The building on the north side of Madison is Michael Graves's 1982 postmodern Portland Building, once considered very controversial because of its radical design. The teal-colored tiles and decorative accents give it the appearance of a giant birthday gift.

To your left is the sandstone Portland City Hall, renovated in 1998. As you walk south past the building, note the Liberty Bell reproduction in the courtyard. When a 1970 bomb damaged the original replica, along with City Hall, the people of Philadelphia gave this replacement to Portland schoolchildren. Many Portland photographs, paintings, tiles, and sculptures can be found inside the building.

▸Turn right on Jefferson and continue along the south side of City Hall to 5th. Look right to view the front entrance incorporating classical Roman balustrades, Tuscan columns, and a dominant rotunda. Every Portland civic building displays a different style of architecture.

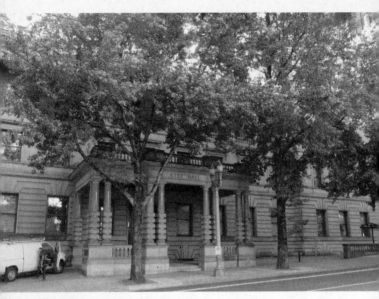

City Hall is still in use. *Dick Lukins*

▸Turn left on 5th, cross Jefferson, and walk past Portland's tallest building, the Wells Fargo Bank Tower, "designed like a rocket to challenge Mount Hood." On the west side of 5th is the Unitus Plaza building. Formerly the Hoffman Columbia Plaza, Pietro Belluschi designed this on a scale to complement City Hall.

▸Cross Columbia. Engraved into the red granite walls of the 500 Building is a sign referring to this as BEGIN AGAIN CORNER. The verses on both sides of this corner are from a poem by Kim Stafford, a local poet and professor. The swordtail fern decorations are by Anne Storrs.

▶Turn east on Columbia and cross 4th. Turn south one block. Cross Clay and turn left on the walkway onto the upper level of the Ira C. Keller Memorial Fountain. This whole city block is a favorite summer play place for Portland youngsters, and adults. The shady ponds on the upper concrete terraces, together with cascading water-falls pooling around the stepping-stones at the lower level, represent mountains, streams, and other kinds of moving water. Sometimes called "Ira's Fountain," it is the highest man-made waterfall in Oregon.

▶Descend the ramp, or take some optional side steps on your right that go down to a small alcove next to the waterfall. Exit the sidewalk at 3rd and Clay. Diagonally opposite is the KOIN Center, a redbrick tower shaped like a fat kindergarten crayon with a big blue point. A tele-vision station and other offices are located on the lower floors, while luxury apartments fill the upper levels.

Straight across on the east side of 3rd is the front entrance of the Portland Civic Auditorium, home of the Portland Opera and Oregon Ballet Theatre, and host of many traveling Broadway shows.

▶Turn south in front of the fountain to Market Street. Turn right and take the path up on the other side of the fountain to 4th Avenue. Then turn left and cross Market Street.

▶Pass the AT&T Market Center building and stop at the Mill Street walkway. This is the west edge of the Portland Center urban renewal project. Thirty-six blocks were razed in the 1950s to create this "New Town" of office buildings, parks, and high-rise apartments, and the apartment buildings are still popular some sixty years later. The original street layout was kept, although many streets became pedestrian walkways. Mill Street is one of these. Diagonally across 4th from the former Mill Street is the Church of Saint Michael the Archangel. Built as a German cathedral, it later became the Italian National Church at the center of the surrounding Italian neighborhood. It's still Roman Catholic, even though urban renewal forced out many original parishioners.

▶Turn left onto the Mill Street walkway and go to the T intersection at the wall with a yellow metal sculpture named *Awning*. This walkway is the pedestrian continuation of 3rd Avenue.

▶Turn right here and take the first walkway on your left into Pettygrove Park. Named for Francis Pettygrove, whose coin toss won him the right to name Portland after his native state's capital, its grassy mounds make the park seem larger than it is, and earned it the nickname of "Mae West Park."

▶Continue along the walkway, angling right to Manuel Izquierdo's *The Dreamer,* a large golden-bronze sculpture surrounded by a pool. When it rains, the urethane foam filler softens the sound of the raindrops hitting the statue.

▶Beyond *The Dreamer,* head south on the walkway between high-rise apartments and office buildings, to the wooden posts marking Harrison Street.

▶Cross Harrison cautiously between these posts and continue south until you see another similarly sized park on your right named for Asa Lovejoy. He lost the historic coin toss with Pettygrove that decided Portland's name. The same coin, now in the Oregon Historical Society, was tossed again to decide which of the two parks would have which name. Lovejoy Park was once described by author Terence O'Donnell as "an origami in concrete." It contains a picnic pavilion and a fountain that "captures the spirit of Oregon streams" as it cascades over steps and terraces into a small pool at the base.

▶Continue south on the walkway past the park until you spot the small brick fountain known as The Chimney. This is the southern edge of the New Town development.

▶Pass the fountain, go to Lincoln Street, and turn right. On your right is the apartment complex, the Village at Lovejoy Fountain, the first building to mix lower-income apartments with market-rate. Pass by and turn right between wooden posts on the next walkway. The Village's swimming pool and courtyard are on your right.

▶Pass by the first walkway on the left, and take the second left-hand walkway up to the plaza by Portland State University's Engineering School on 4th Avenue. The large steel structure flying overhead is named *Tecotosh*.

▶Turn right on 4th and walk to the traffic signal at Hall Street.

▶Turn left on Hall, cross 4th, and go west one block to 5th Avenue. Across 5th is a huge acrylic painting of book spines covering most of the building facing you. This art piece is called *The Knowledge,* and the books pictured are all found in PSU's Millar Library.

▶Cross 5th and continue to 6th. Cross. Turn right, crossing Hall. Twelve granite sculptures sit on the grassy verges along the street here, all part of Fernanda D'Agostino's *Urban Hydrology.*

▶Cross 6th Avenue and turn north. Look closely at the etchings on the black squares, *Patterns May Be an Action or the Trace Left by an Action,* on Parking Garage #1. This art is also by Fernanda D'Agostino.

▶Cross Harrison. Pass by the School of Business to the small park at the corner of 6th and Montgomery. Look left to the sign giving information about this Permaculture Park, with a variety of sustainable plants requiring little care. Note Electric Avenue, with its charging stations for electric cars and electric bicycles.

▶Cross 6th at Montgomery. Ahead is Portland State University's Urban Transit Center, where the MAX train and the streetcar meet. This side of the plaza is the start of a rectilinear water feature, where water flows from one man-made trough to another, to the 5th Street Plaza. Descend to find cafes, the PSU bookstore, more running water, and monoliths casting granite shadows.

▶Walk north at the center of the 5th Street Plaza and exit at 6th and Mill. Turn right on 6th crossing Mill Street, then Market. Cross Clay and note the five parts of Michihiro

Kosuge's sculpture group, *Continuation,* with some pieces installed in a restaurant courtyard.

▶Still on 6th Avenue, cross Columbia and Jefferson. Look across 6th to view the University Club. The Jacobean-style facade resembles college buildings in England and on the East Coast. Two similar apartment houses nearby give a glimpse of an earlier gracious world.

▶Continue north on 6th and cross Madison Street. Look west to see Tom Hardy's sculpture, *Running Horses,* in front of the Gus Solomon US Courthouse, a limestone building with terra-cotta decorations. It was formerly mounted at Pioneer Plaza.

▶The Standard Plaza fills the block on your right. In front of this building is *The Ring of Time,* a rough metal sculpture shaped like a giant Möbius strip.

▶Go across the bridge to the entrance door. The bridge crosses above a lovely courtyard with leaf-covered walls and two circular fountains lined with turquoise mosaic tiles.

▶If the Standard building is open, enter the front lobby. Pass the information desk to go through the glass doors to the 5th Avenue side. Here, you'll get a spectacular view of the Portland Building and *Portlandia.* You are almost on the same level as the statue. The 38-foot figure of *Portlandia* is made of hammered copper sheeting over a steel armature—the same method used in making the *Statue of Liberty.* Her image was adapted from an old Portland city seal. Leave the lobby by taking the escalator down to street

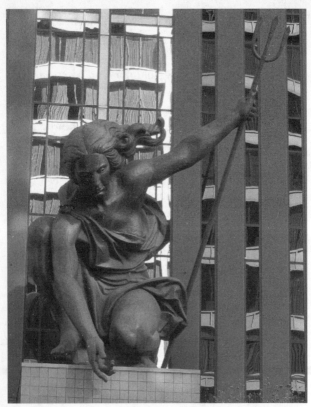

This massive copper sculpture is a Portland icon. *Dick Lukins*

level, exiting to the 5th Avenue Plaza. (If the building was closed, return to 6th and take the ramp by Main Street down into the lower courtyard, exiting on 5th Avenue. Turn right to the plaza in front of the building.) From this plaza, you will get another good view of *Portlandia.* A sign displays a verse from the prize-winning "Ode to

Portlandia," as well as some of the statue's statistics and history.

▸Main Street is on your left. Cross it and go north on 5th to Salmon, passing the concrete Multnomah County Courthouse across 5th. This has been in use for over a century. Originally, the building had a central courtyard, where Prohibition-era confiscated alcohol was poured down a drain.

▸Cross Salmon. Continue straight to Taylor Street. Across 5th Avenue to your right is a large marble fountain by sculptor Count Alexander von Svoboda. Officially entitled *The Quest,* it is sometimes referred to as "Three Groins in the Fountain."

▸Turn left onto Taylor. Go one block west to 6th Avenue.

▸Cross 6th to the corner of the Hilton Hotel.

▸Cross Yamhill and return to your starting point at Pioneer Courthouse Square.

Walk 3: The Cultural District

◻ ✕ 🛒 👫 🏢 ♿

General location: The Portland Cultural Center is part of downtown Portland, just west of I-5.

Special attractions: Theaters, music, museums, indoor and outdoor art, varied architecture, and the Portland State University campus

Difficulty: Easy, flat; entirely on paved sidewalk with curb cuts, and the entire walk is wheelchair-accessible

Distance: 3.25 miles

Estimated time: 1.5 hours

Services: Restrooms are located inside the TriMet offices in Pioneer Courthouse Square and in all public buildings. Stores and restaurants are located throughout the area.

Restrictions: The Portland Visitor Information Center and TriMet information center are open Monday through Friday, 8:30 a.m. to 5:30 p.m.; Saturday, 10 a.m. to 4 p.m.; Sunday, 10 a.m. to 2 p.m. (May through October only). The restrooms are open every day from 8 a.m. to 7 p.m. Most public buildings have wheelchair-accessible restrooms and are open weekdays from 9 a.m. to 5 p.m.

For more information: Contact the Portland Oregon Visitors Association.

Getting started: This walk begins at Pioneer Courthouse Square, between Broadway and 6th Avenues and Morrison and Yamhill Streets. From I-5 northbound, take the exit to I-405, then take the 6th Avenue exit and go south to Yamhill Street and Pioneer Courthouse Square. From US 26 eastbound, take the Market Street exit and follow the City

Center signs to 10th Avenue. Turn left onto 10th, cross Taylor Street, and turn right onto Yamhill. Go three blocks.

There are three "Smart Park" parking garages in the immediate vicinity. One is on 10th between Morrison and Yamhill, one is at 3rd Avenue and Alder Street, and one is at 4th and Yamhill. These city garages offer the cheapest parking in town. Look for the red "Smart Park" signs.

Public transportation: Buses, the Portland Streetcar, and MAX light-rail lines meet at Pioneer Courthouse Square. Contact TriMet for information about fares and schedules (trimet.org).

Overview: This walk begins at the central plaza of downtown Portland, easily reached on foot from most downtown hotels. This square, scene of countless festivals and outdoor exhibits, is bordered by department stores, specialty shops within reconstructed buildings, excellent restaurants, and one-of-a-kind boutiques. The walk continues through twelve tree-shaded Park Blocks, passing the Multnomah County Library, the Oregon History Center, the Center for the Performing Arts, the Portland Art Museum, and the campus of Portland State University.

The Walk

▶Start this walk at the Morrison Street and Broadway corner of Pioneer Courthouse Square, near Starbucks.

▶Cross Broadway and turn right to cross Morrison. Continue two blocks north to Washington Street. Cross Washington and turn left one block to Park. Cross.

The park to your right is O'Bryant Square, named for the mayor who founded Portland's first public library. This

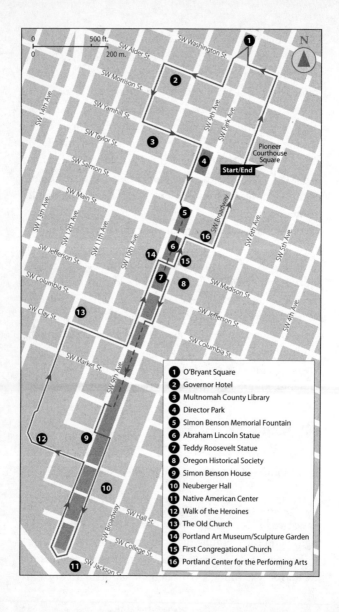

1	O'Bryant Square
2	Governor Hotel
3	Multnomah County Library
4	Director Park
5	Simon Benson Memorial Fountain
6	Abraham Lincoln Statue
7	Teddy Roosevelt Statue
8	Oregon Historical Society
9	Simon Benson House
10	Neuberger Hall
11	Native American Center
12	Walk of the Heroines
13	The Old Church
14	Portland Art Museum/Sculpture Garden
15	First Congregational Church
16	Portland Center for the Performing Arts

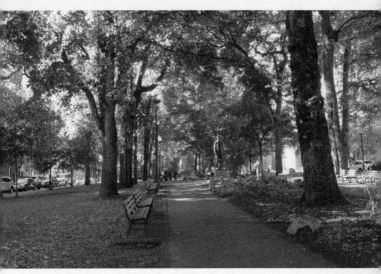

This view looks north on the South Park Blocks. *Dick Lukins*

is one of the early Park Blocks, planned to run through the city from north to south. This urban plaza park is also the first one in Portland built on top of an underground parking garage, so it has less greenery than most parks. Note the large "fountain for a rose" at the northeast end, with a bronze sign explaining who was the donor and why.

▶Turn left at 9th Avenue and go one block south to Alder. Turn right on Alder. Cross 9th, passing a parking lot, host to one of Portland's large collection of food carts. You can find a wide variety of international flavors here, from Egyptian to Korean fusion. Look across to admire the terra-cotta ornamentation on the facade of the Governor Hotel. Originally the 1909 Seward Hotel, this has long been a popular meeting site for Portland's businessmen.

Jake's Grill still displays the original dark woodwork and stuffed animal heads inside.

▸Cross 10th and go past the hotel to 11th. Turn left. This terra-cotta structure with a classical Greek facade was first built as an Elks Temple, and later became the Princeton Club. Now it's the west side of the Governor Hotel.

▸Proceed two blocks to Yamhill and cross to the northwest corner of the venerable Multnomah County Library, which fills the entire block. Names of various topics and subject disciplines found inside the library are inscribed at the top of the building. These include fine arts, engineering, science, history, and philology, among others.

▸Turn east along the north side of the library. Architect A. E. Doyle used benches to disguise the slope of the lot as it goes downhill to 10th. Named after classic authors, they provide pleasant places to rest and read along the sidewalk.

▸Stop at the third bench, dedicated to Robert Louis Stevenson. Across Yamhill you can see Number 1023, the building that once housed Louise Bryant's studio. She was the artist who accompanied Portland-born journalist John Reed (the subject of the 1981 film, *Reds*) to Moscow when he covered the beginnings of the Russian Revolution.

MULTNOMAH COUNTY LIBRARY

This timeless, classically designed building may be one of architect A. E. Doyle's most famous structures.

It was completely renovated in 1997. Doyle's grandson, George McMath, was one of the architects who worked on this renovation. The classic exterior remains much the same, but the interior walls were completely rebuilt. Most of the original decorations, columns, and wainscoting were retained.

The entrance is on 10th Avenue. The inside theme, "Garden of Knowledge," came from the names of the thinkers and authors inscribed on the exterior of the library, and from the surrounding tall trees. It is reflected in the overhead garland adorning the lobby foyer, the leaves etched into the steps of the grand staircase, and a wreath encircling the second-floor lighting fixture. The Beverly Cleary Children's Room has a delightful bronze tree in its center, with all sorts of sculpted natural-history objects hidden in the trunk. A sculpture of the artist's dog sits at the base of the tree.

▶Continue on Yamhill. Cross 10th at the traffic signals, and go one block east to 9th. Cross 9th Avenue into Director Park, one of the "missing park blocks." Developer Thomas P. Moyer planned a twelve-story parking garage here, but later agreed to let the space revert to its original purpose as a park block. It took leadership as well as funding by Moyer, Jordan Schnitzer, and other donors to work with city planners and create this pleasant urban plaza over a huge subterranean parking garage.

Chess players are attracted to the southern section with its small chessboards and the large one inlaid among the pavers. The park hosts often bring out giant plastic chessmen to use in a life-size game. Chairs and tables can be moved to sunny spots where you can listen to water flowing and children's chatter as they wade in the Teachers Fountain. The public art piece suspended from the high canopy becomes "an abstract, striated tapestry of light and color" after dark.

▸Return to 9th. Cross Taylor and proceed south to Salmon Street. You are at the corner of the Arlington Club, once a private and exclusive club for Portland's influential men. At Salmon, 9th Avenue changes its name to Park Avenue, the same as the street running along the other side of the Park Blocks.

▸Cross Salmon. On this side of the street, opposite the Arlington Club, is the Simon Benson Memorial Fountain, designed by A. E. Doyle in honor of the donor of the first Benson Bubbler drinking fountains.

▸Take the wide curb cut to enter the South Park Blocks. This is often referred to as Shemanski Park in honor of the donor of the fountain with its low drinking bowls for pets. Joseph Shemanski gave this to the city in 1926, to "express in small measure gratitude for what the city has done for me." *Rebecca at the Well* symbolizes welcome, since the biblical Rebecca was noted for her hospitality and kindness to strangers and animals.

▸Before crossing Main Street, look to your left. The building across Park Avenue is the Arlene Schnitzer Concert Hall, part of the Portland Center for the Performing Arts.

▸Continue straight across Main, keeping on the center walkway in the park block. Look left across Park to

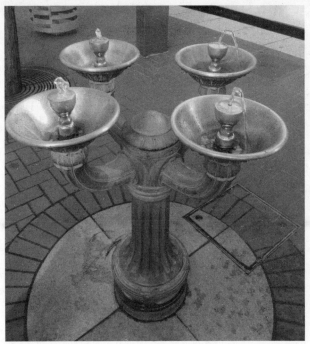

A Benson Bubbler offers a cool drink. *Dick Lukins*

better observe the First Congregational Church's distinctive basalt and limestone walls. From here, you can see how well the lines of the Antoinette Hatfield Hall blend with those of the church walls.

▶Then keep on the center parkway toward the bronze statue of Abraham Lincoln. It has been criticized as being too melancholy, but sculptor George Fite Waters (a pupil of Rodin's) said this was how Lincoln looked during the Civil War. It was donated by Dr. Henry Waldo Coe.

▸Cross Madison Street and go to the Theodore Roosevelt statue, also donated by Dr. Coe. Coe began practicing medicine in North Dakota in the 1880s, and became one of Roosevelt's hunting companions before moving to Portland. For this statue of his old friend, he chose well-known sculptor Alexander Phimister Proctor. The bronze tablet at the base contains a wonderful tribute to the president.

▸Walk to the plaque at Jefferson Street. This marks the location of Portland's earliest planked road, allowing produce and goods to be hauled back and forth to the fertile valley beyond the Tualatin (now West) hills.

▸Return to the Roosevelt statue. Look east across Park Avenue. The side of the Oregon History Center looks so three-dimensional that you would swear it was carved from stone. Richard Haas created the eight-story trompe l'oeil murals that are on two sides of the Oregon History Center. The mural on the front side of the building shows members of the Lewis and Clark Expedition. If you look closely, you can see Meriwether Lewis, the slave York, Sacagawea with her baby, Jean Baptiste, and Lewis's dog Seaman. The dog is 7 feet tall, giving you some idea of the size of the murals.

▸Cross Park Avenue to the building, headquarters of the Oregon Historical Society. You can enter the "Washington Ellipse" courtyard by the steps or by the wheelchair ramp. The large sculpture, *Flying Together*, is by Tom Hardy. Inside are interactive exhibits, informative displays about Oregon history (including the coin used to determine Portland's name), and an extensive research library.

►Come out of the courtyard, turn south on Park Avenue, cross Jefferson, and go to Columbia. On this northeast corner of Columbia and Park is the First Christian Church. This is the only Portland congregation still worshipping in a building on its original site, though the present building dates from 1919.

►Cross Columbia, turn right, and cross back into the Park Blocks.

►Keep on the center walk, passing the three large stone blocks on the ground named *Peace Chant*. Cross Market Street and you will be on the Portland State University Campus. It was started as an extension center for returning veterans in the Vanport housing project for shipyard workers. When the entire area was wiped out in the 1948 Columbia flood, the college relocated to the Lincoln High School Building, now Lincoln Hall.

►Turn right on the Mill Street walkway and go west. Turn left (south), passing the Vue Apartments with their little waterfall, and go to the Queen Anne house on the corner of Montgomery and Park.

This elegant mansion was abandoned and in disrepair on nearby Clay Street until a small group, the Friends of the Simon Benson House, managed to raise enough funds to move the house in 2000 from its original location to this spot on the Portland State University campus, where it could be restored and cared for. Simon Benson gave twenty bronze Benson Bubblers to the city to keep his workers sober, so one is now installed in the front yard.

►Go east on the Montgomery Street walkway, passing the fountain, *Farewell to Orpheus,* designed by former PSU art professor, Frederic Littman.

►Turn south on Park, passing the Smith Student Union. Publicly funded works of indoor and outdoor art enhance nearly every building at PSU. One of these, a mural commemorating the Vanport, is located in the second-floor stairwell of this building. There is also a small art gallery.

►Continue south to Neuberger Hall. Tom Hardy's bronze sculpture, *Oregon Country,* screens all the ground-floor windows. Intertwined ships, sand dollars, crabs, and plants represent Oregon's natural history.

►Continue past Shattuck Hall and the tennis courts to the Native American Student and Community Center at SW Jackson Street. Go down the stairs into the little garden at the west end. Look up to see the sculpture called *Salmon Cycle Marker,* way above the garden area.

If the building is open, go in, taking the main hall to the end. Here is a wonderful room, used for many student events. Look through the windows of the drumming circle to see a full-length statue of Chief Joseph, and also admire the many statues and artwork on display.

►Exit on Jackson, turn left, and return to the last Park Block. This is now a children's play park. Take the western side of this block back toward the PSU entrance, passing the Scott Center and the Millar Library. Look right to see the limestone sculpture, *Holon.* Turn left on the Harrison Street walkway on the north side of the library.

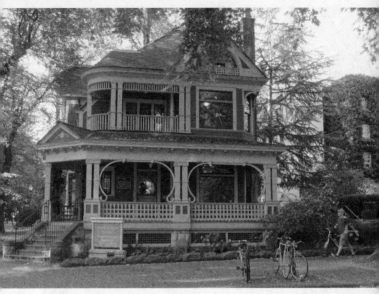

This house belonged to the lumber baron who installed the
first "Benson Bubblers." *Dick Lukins*

▶Continue straight ahead (west) to the end of the walkway
at Hoffman Hall on 11th Avenue. This little park is "the
walk of the heroines," dedicated to the Portland women
who "illuminated our lives." On the granite wall to the left
are the engraved names of many well-known and not-so-
well-known women who gave Portland much of its cultural heritage. A variety of historical quotes about women
are engraved on the walk.

▶Turn right on 11th and go north to Mill Street. On your
left is an interesting art piece at the entrance to the Joseph
C. Blumer Center. *Cobbletale*—created from old streetcar

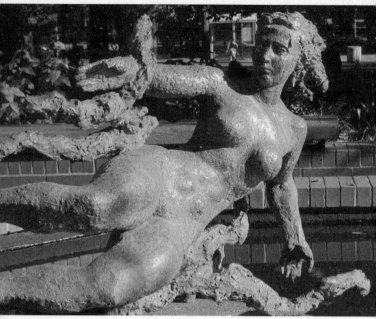

Farewell to Orpheus was designed by one of PSU's own.
Dick Lukins

rails, cobblestones, chunks of concrete, and other pieces of old city streets—rises from the sidewalk in front.

▶Continue on 11th, cross Mill, and continue north, exiting the PSU campus at Market Street. Cross.

▶Stay on the west side of 11th for one block to Clay Street. Diagonally across Clay Street, The Old Church stands on the opposite corner. This is a beautiful and interesting example of Carpenter Gothic. Early Oregon had more woodworkers than masons, so wood was often used to imitate stone. A group of Portland citizens saved this church building from destruction. It's now used as a site for plays, weddings, and a public meeting place.

▶Turn right on Clay for two blocks. Cross 11th, and then 10th.

▶On your right is the South Park Square apartment complex. Notice the trees etched into its brick wall.

▶When you reach Park Avenue, turn left, cross Clay, and continue north for one block to Columbia Street. Cross. If you are observant, you will spy a small sculpture called

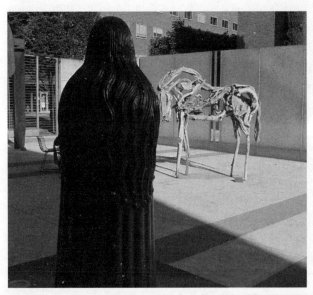

Madrina and *Horse* are two works of art found in the Sculpture Courtyard. *Dick Lukins*

From Within, Shalom, located in front of the St. James Lutheran Church. This echoes the *Peace Chant* sculpture of the three stone slabs in this section of the Park Block across the street.

▶Continue to Jefferson Street and cross, continuing to the entrance of the Portland Art Museum. This award-winning 1930 building was designed by Pietro Belluschi, the architect of many buildings in Portland. Pass the museum and turn left into the outdoor sculpture court. A wide assortment of large museum pieces are here, ranging from Roy Lichtenstein's *Brushstrokes* to Mel Katz's scarlet *Garden Gate,* resembling a Chinese character, to Mark Calderon's *Madrina,* a woman looking the same from all sides. The Portland Art Museum's Mark Building, formerly the Masonic Temple, is on the north side of the courtyard. The Masons supposedly modeled this temple on biblical descriptions of the one built by King Solomon.

▶Return to West Park. Cross the Park Blocks to the First Congregational United Church of Christ on the corner of Madison and East Park Avenue. Modeled after Boston's Old South Church, it was built in 1890. Many Portland citizens disliked this Italian Gothic structure when it was first built, and the dark basalt and light limestone pattern inspired the nickname, Holy Checkerboard. Only the white tower remains. This is the only downtown church with a bell still in use.

▶Turn left (north) on East Park, and then turn right on Main Street.

▶Continue straight ahead on Main for one block, to Broadway. You are skirting the south side of the Arlene Schnitzer Concert Hall. At the corner of Broadway and Main is the original canopy and sign for the old Portland Theater. Look to your right for the Antoinette Hatfield Hall, part of the Portland Center for the Performing Arts. Turn left on Broadway to the well-known Heathman Hotel just ahead before crossing Salmon.

▶Follow Broadway south for two blocks to Yamhill. From here, look across Yamhill for a good view of the Jackson Tower. It has been lighting up the Portland skyline since its construction in 1912. Outlining the building are 1,800 light sockets, which were built into the original terra-cotta. When the building was originally constructed to house the *Oregon Journal,* the large clocks in the tower chimed every fifteen minutes.

▶Cross Yamhill and return to your starting point in Pioneer Courthouse Square.

Walk 4: The Pearl and Chinatown

✗ 🛒 👪 🏢 ♿

General location: Downtown Portland, west of I-5

Special attractions: Powell's Books, the Chinese Garden, the Nikkei Legacy Center, galleries, restaurants, and shops

Difficulty: Easy, flat; entirely on paved sidewalks

Distance: 3 miles

Estimated time: 2 hours

Services: Restrooms are located inside the TriMet offices in Pioneer Courthouse Square and in all public buildings. Stores and restaurants are located throughout the area.

Restrictions: The Portland Visitor Information Center and TriMet information center are open Monday through Friday, 8:30 a.m. to 5:30 p.m.; Saturday, 10 a.m. to 4 p.m.; Sunday, 10 a.m. to 2 p.m. (May through October only). The restrooms are open every day from 8 a.m. to 7 p.m. Most public buildings have wheelchair-accessible restrooms and are open weekdays from 9 a.m. to 5 p.m.

For more information: Contact the Portland Oregon Visitors Association.

Getting started: This walk begins at Pioneer Courthouse Square, between Broadway and 6th Avenues and Morrison and Yamhill Streets. From I-5 northbound, take the exit to I-405, then take the 6th Avenue exit and go south to Yamhill Street and Pioneer Courthouse Square. From US 26 eastbound, take the Market Street exit and follow the City Center signs to 10th Avenue. Turn left onto 10th, cross Taylor Street, and turn right onto Yamhill. Go three blocks.

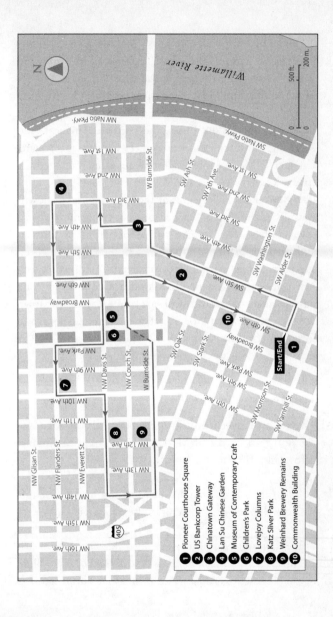

N

Willamette River

NW Natio Pkwy.

SW Natio Prwy.

NW 1st Ave.

W Burnside St.

NW 2nd Ave.

SW Ash St.

SW 2nd Ave.

SW 5th Ave.

SW 1st Ave.

NW 3rd Ave.

SW 3rd Ave.

SW 2nd Ave.

SW Washington St.

SW 4th Ave.

NW 4th Ave.

NW 5th Ave.

SW Alder St.

NW 6th Ave.

SW 5th Ave.

NW Broadway

SW 6th Ave.

SW Broadway

NW Park Ave.

SW Oak St.

SW Stark St.

NW 9th Ave.

SW Park Ave.

NW Davis St.

NW Couch St.

W Burnside St.

SW 9th Ave.

SW 10th Ave.

SW Morrison St.

SW Yamhill St.

NW 10th Ave.

NW 11th Ave.

NW 12th Ave.

NW 13th Ave.

NW Glisan St.

NW Flanders St.

NW Everett St.

NW 14th Ave.

NW 15th Ave.

NW 16th Ave.

405

Start/End

1 Pioneer Courthouse Square
2 US Bankcorp Tower
3 Chinatown Gateway
4 Lan Su Chinese Garden
5 Museum of Contemporary Craft
6 Children's Park
7 Lovejoy Columns
8 Katz Silver Park
9 Weinhard Brewery Remains
10 Commonwealth Building

500 ft.

200 m.

There are three "Smart Park" parking garages in the immediate vicinity. One is on 10th between Morrison and Yamhill, one is at 3rd Avenue and Alder Street, and one is at 4th and Yamhill. These city garages offer the cheapest parking in town. Look for the red "Smart Park" signs.

Public transportation: Buses, the Portland Streetcar, and MAX light-rail lines meet at Pioneer Courthouse Square. Contact TriMet for information about fares and schedules (trimet.org).

Overview: This walk begins at the central plaza of downtown Portland, easily reached on foot from most downtown hotels. This square, scene of countless festivals and outdoor exhibits, is bordered by department stores, specialty shops within reconstructed buildings, excellent restaurants, and one-of-a-kind boutiques. The walk passes much of the sidewalk art around the downtown transit malls. You will see art galleries, antiques shops, and interior-decorating stores in the Pearl District, as well as experience Chinatown's unique ambience.

The Walk

▶Begin at Pioneer Courthouse Square. Exit the square at the northeast corner of Morrison Street and 6th Avenue, across from the Pioneer Courthouse.

▶Cross 6th and go straight on Morrison to 5th Avenue. Pass the *Animals in Pools* sculptures by Georgia Gerber.

▶Turn left and cross Morrison onto the west side of 5th Avenue. Pass *Whistlestop for an Organ Teacher,* resembling organ pipes. Cross Alder to see *Interlocking Forms,* another limestone sculpture, then cross Washington. Note the large bronze *Floribunda,* resembling an abstract topknot, just before reaching Stark.

▶As you cross Stark, you can smell the stationary food carts on the east side of 5th. Each sells a different freshly prepared food. Notice the signs on the curb side of the sidewalk in front of the booths. These are not posters but laminated glass works called *Reading the Street,* with silhouetted figures changing in the light.

▶At Oak, cross 5th Avenue and continue north. The bright crayon colors of John Killmaster's untitled porcelain enamel piece make it resemble a child's building set. Another different but colorful untitled piece on the north side of Pine is by Ivan Morrison. The panels form a child-size hiding place.

▶Continue to the large brick plaza at Burnside Street and the large, tubular, metal fountain nicknamed "The Car Wash." The fountain is turned off on really windy days to protect passing pedestrians from the spray. US Bancorp Tower, a Portland landmark frequently referred to as "Big Pink," is across 5th. The Portland City Grill on the thirtieth floor offers marvelous views of the city.

▶Turn right on Burnside for one block. Cross Burnside at 4th, and enter the Chinatown District through the *Chinatown Gate.* This authentic reproduction of ancient Chinese gates was dedicated in 1986. English and Chinese signs on each marble pillar give the information about this gift to Portland. On either side are large stone and porcelain

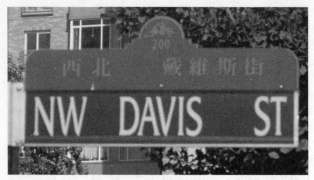

Bilingual signs guide you in English and Chinese. *Dick Lukins*

lions. Look up to see the five roofs and count sixty-four gold dragons.

▶Cross 4th and take the sidewalk on the right side. Walk north. Red lampposts and signposts brighten the area and cherry trees line the streets, especially beautiful in springtime. There are two street signs on every signpost: one in English, and one in Chinese.

▶Continue for one block to Couch Street. Cross. Look for the bronze plaque in the pavement outside the former Hung Far Low Restaurant. Embossed with a flower and a persimmon, it gives a bit of the restaurant history.

▶Continue to Davis Street. Across Davis is the House of Louie, decorated with Chinese motifs.

▶Turn right on the corridor between the two red granite *Festival Lanterns* by Brian Goldbloom. Under each are replica artifacts from the days when the Chinese were brought

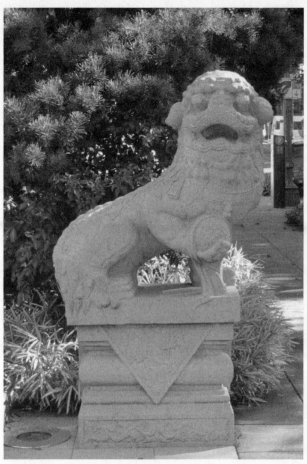

One of the guardian lions (Foo Dogs) protects Lan Su.

Dick Lukins

here as laborers. Exit to 3rd Avenue between two more
Festival Lanterns in black steel and granite. Different sets
of artifacts are underneath.

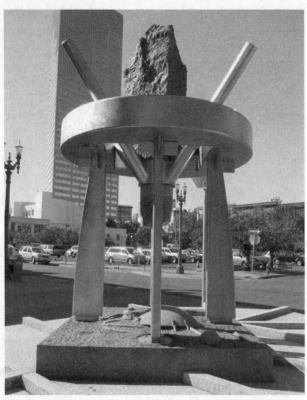

Each base of the Festival Lanterns displays different artifacts representing Chinese labor. *Dick Lukins*

▶Cross 3rd and turn left. Proceed to Everett and cross. You are at the entrance courtyard of the Lan Su Chinese Garden, a reproduction of a Ming Dynasty (1368–1644) scholar's garden. Opened in 2000, its white walls enclose an entire city block formerly used for parking.

LAN SU CHINESE GARDEN

"Lan Su" is a combination of syllables from Suzhou, China (one of Portland's sister cities), and Portland, and the Chinese characters mean "Garden of the Awakening Orchids." Most of the materials, including the Lake Tai rock, came from China. This rock is both yin and yang (hard and soft), since the hard rock is sculpted and then put back in the lake to soften. The American landscape architect designed the overall plans and elevations for the site and then worked

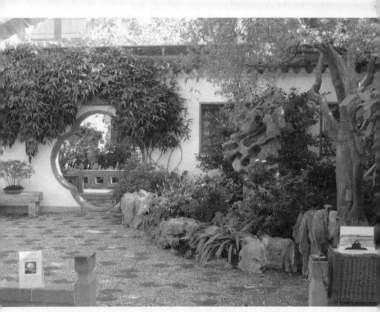

Entry into the Classical Chinese Garden. *Dick Lukins*

with a landscape architect trained in Chinese garden design, who, being Chinese-born, could communicate with the sixty-five artisans sent over from Suzhou.

It is amazing how several buildings, a climbable hill, and a small lake can give the impression of a large countryside in one city block. Pay the small entrance fee and you will feel far away from the city's hustle and bustle. It is designed to appeal to the senses of touch, smell, sight, and hearing, at all seasons of the year, and the teahouse also appeals with scents and tastes. Chinese artifacts and garden plants are for sale in the gift shop and inside the entrance courtyard.

▶Leave the courtyard and continue north on 3rd. Walk one more block to Flanders, cross 3rd, and take the walkway between two more black steel-and-granite *Festival Lanterns*. Pass the final set of red ones on 4th.

▶Continue two blocks straight west on Flanders and turn left on 6th Avenue for two blocks, toward Davis. Cross Davis. In the middle of this block is a small obelisk topped with a green man. Artist Daniel Duford has changed the English "bronze figure" legend into one about a Portland phantom who shoots invisible arrows at passersby. Those who are touched find the invisible world made visible, sometimes even seeing a white stag stalking the night sky. The tale is told in two statues and eight display signs on 5th and 6th Streets, between Burnside and Glisan. If curious, find them all—in any order—to visualize a complete story before returning to Davis Street.

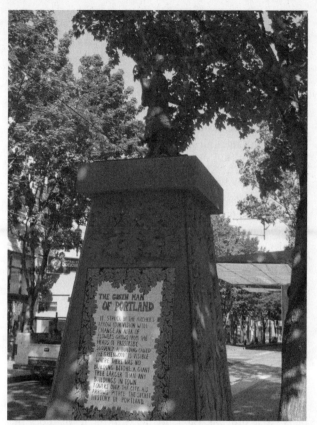

The "Green Man" is an an adaptation of a British legend.

Dick Lukins

▶Turn west on Davis and go one block to Broadway. This street separates Chinatown from the Pearl District, an area known for its many interesting art galleries and shops. Cross Broadway and proceed on Davis to see the Museum of Contemporary Craft, a very successful Works Progress Administration

(WPA) project that has helped Oregon craftsmen for almost seventy-five years. It has recently become part of the Pacific Northwest College of Art (PNCA). Their sales gallery, open to the public, represents artists in ceramics, glass, jewelry, wood, metal, fiber, and mixed media. In 2015 the PNCA has plans to renovate the former 511 Broadway federal building a few blocks north, relocating scattered classrooms into one building and utilizing the blocks as an outdoor campus.

▶Cross 8th into the North Park Blocks. Captain John Couch donated this part of his land claim as a park, continuing the layout of the South Park Blocks. The lovely old elms arching overhead are among the few that survived an epidemic of Dutch elm disease. One of the oldest children's parks is in the block on your left. Originally, boys and girls were segregated here into two separate play areas, with supervisors making sure the sexes didn't mix. Now everyone plays together.

▶Go to the sidewalk on the west side of the park, cross Davis, and turn north to find William Wegman's *Dog Bowl*. Wegman, well known for his dog greeting cards and calendars, doesn't consider this battered-looking bowl an "art" installation. However, like Simon Benson's "bubblers" that provide water for his workmen, this does the same for pets.

▶Continue on the walkway, crossing Everett. Turn left on Flanders, crossing Park and 9th Avenues, and stop on 10th.

▶Turn left and walk a few steps to a small plaza containing the remnants of two support columns for a bridge over the nearby railroad yards. These are the *Lovejoy Columns*, scrawled by Tom Stefopoulos, an immigrant Greek artist, while working as a railway watchman. When the yards were demolished, an outcry from local artists convinced city officials these charcoal drawings were folk art, not graffiti, and should be saved. So here they are, surrounded by upscale shops and condos.

▶Exit the plaza on 10th and turn south two blocks to Davis. Stop at the corner and look across for a good view of the redbrick building with castle-like architecture. This is the former armory, now the Gerding Theater, and home to Portland Center Stage.

▶Cross Davis and turn right. Alongside the theater building is a "sliver park" named for former mayor Vera Katz. You can read a bit about her on the surrounding walls, made of stone matching the original armory foundations. The park combines plants and a water feature and blends in totally with its surroundings.

▶Cross 11th and continue to 14th Avenue. A storage building on your right is decorated with Virginia Flynn's *Pearl Vignettes* on the corner walls. Silhouettes portray active people in this district: bicyclists, diners, musicians, walkers, and drivers of different vehicles.

▶Turn left on 14th Avenue and walk two blocks to Burnside. Turn left and cross 13th. On the opposite side you can see the *People's Bike Library,* a sculpture made entirely of old bikes, and topped with one painted in gleaming gold.

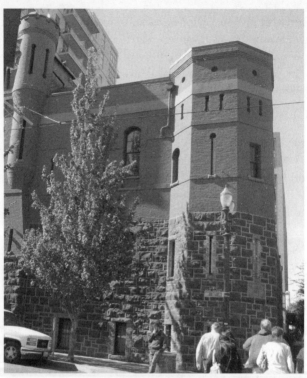

This former armory is now the Gerding Theater. *Dick Lukins*

▶Continue east on Burnside for one block, to 12th. Two original walls of the 1860 Henry Weinhard brewery still remain on the north side. The building is now the Brewery Lofts, a trendy apartment building. Henry's Pub has replaced the original brewery tasting room.

▶Cross 12th and 11th to Powell's Books. This famous independent bookstore fills a city block. If you enter, pick up a bookstore map before navigating the 43,000-square-foot rabbit hole containing half a million books. Different subjects are arranged in rooms of different colors, and enthusiastic staff members will help you find just what you are looking for. You can snack in the small coffee shop while reading available magazines and newspapers. If you enter the store, make sure you take the exit to Burnside (it's easy to get confused).

At the corner of Burnside and 10th, on the traffic island where Oak comes in at an angle, is Peter Beeman's giant *Pod*. A cluster of wires jutting out on top fan out in a strong wind, or when pedestrians push on the pendulum.

▶Cross 10th and go two blocks east to the Park Avenue entrance to the North Park Blocks. A huge bronze replica of a Shang Dynasty pitcher centers this block. Baby elephant Xi'an Bao rides on the back of his parent, Da Tung.

▶After admiring the elephant, take the East Park walkway to Couch. Looking across Park, you can see the Blue Sky Gallery, founded in 1975 as the Oregon Center for the Photographic Arts. At Couch Street and Eighth is one of Portland's famous "Loos," hygienic public bathrooms designed to serve needs and discourage other uses. Students from nearby Emerson School designed the colorful door, installed in a celebration that featured songs such as "Skip to my 'Loo,'" and a visit from a city commissioner.

▶Cross 8th and continue two blocks on Couch to NW 6th Avenue.

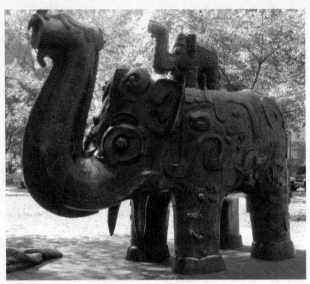

Xi'an Bao rides atop Da Tung. *Dick Lukins*

▶Turn right one block to Burnside. Cross Burnside at the traffic signal to "Big Pink," which fills the block on the east side of the street.

▶Continue on SW 6th Avenue to Pine Street. On your left are three bronze artworks by Bruce Conkle, entitled *Burls Will Be Burls,* representing the water cycle.

▶Cross Pine to watch the sheets of water cascading over Lee Kelly's 20-foot-tall steel structure on the corner of 6th and Pine. This is one of many untitled artworks in Portland that encourage viewers to supply their own interpretations and nicknames.

▶Cross Oak. Pass by John Buck's *Lodge Grass.* As you approach Stark, look across 6th to see a geometric bronze sculpture, *Talus #2,* representing a legendary defender of Crete.

▶Continue on 6th to Stark. Here are some different types of building design. The neoclassical US National Bank Building on your right was built in 1917, with dramatic relief panels on its bronze doors. The 1925 Bank of California building across 6th is an example of the Italian Renaissance style.

▶Cross Stark. Mel Katz's colorful and modern *Daddy Long Legs* is near the corner of the Commonwealth Building, one of the first glass "curtain wall" skyscrapers designed by Pietro Belluschi. You have to look up to get the full impact.

▶Continue to the corner of Washington, cross, and pass by Malia Jensen's bronze sculpture, called *Pile*—a stack of artifacts representing Portland life. These suggest working, home, and communication, with two urban birds on top.

▶Continue across Alder and notice Norman Taylor's bronze female figure, *Kvinneakt,* just before Morrison Street. This Norwegian "nude woman" became famous shortly after her 1975 installation when Bud Clark, later a mayor of Portland, was photographed facing the sculpture with his back to the camera and his raincoat outstretched. The image was reproduced on a famous poster, "Expose Yourself to Art." Some reproductions are featured on notecards sold at the Oregon Historical Society.

▶Cross Morrison. You are back at Pioneer Courthouse Square.

Walk 5: Northwest Alphabet District

✗ 🛒 🏢

General location:
Special attractions: City views, Victorian mansions, unique small restaurants, and trendy boutiques
Difficulty: Moderate, with a few steep uphill sections
Distance: 4 miles
Estimated time: 2.5 hours
Services: Restaurants, restrooms, and water
Restrictions: This walk is not suitable for wheelchairs. Narrow sidewalks, few curb cuts, and uphill sections also make it difficult for strollers.
For more information: Contact the Portland Oregon Visitors Association.
Getting started: The walk starts at the Hotel deLuxe, 729 SW 15th Avenue. To reach the hotel from I-5 northbound, take the exit to I-405 and then take the Salmon Street exit. From I-5 southbound, take exit 302B to I-405, then the Couch-Burnside exit. The hotel parking garage is on 15th Avenue, the south side of Yamhill Street, with unlimited parking if you are staying overnight. Metered parking is available on the street.
Public transportation: The MAX light-rail line stops at the Jeld-Wen Stadium station on 18th Street, between Yamhill and Morrison.
Overview: The Hotel deLuxe was formerly the Mallory Hotel, a favorite downtown hotel for many years. Its decor

is reminiscent of the glory days of Hollywood, but the Driftwood Room is still original. The Alphabet District across Burnside is still referred to as Northwest or Nob Hill by most Portlanders, the "Nob Hill" nickname coming from a grocer who wanted to associate this neighborhood with the well-known San Francisco district. Portland's affluent built large magnificent houses here, patterned on mansions found on the East Coast, or in Europe. These proved difficult to keep up, and after World War I later owners moved out and into large apartment houses being built nearby. Although a great many mansions were torn down, several remain and are listed on the National Register of Historic Places. This walk passes some of these originals, as well as many lovingly restored and maintained smaller homes.

This area has recently been rediscovered as a wonderful place to live, with its remaining old trees and gracious landscaping, and newer owners are sprucing up existing housing rather than replacing it. You will see examples of all of these on your walk. Some streets are filled with little shops and restaurants, giving two of the avenues the nicknames of "Trendy-first" and "Trendy-third."

The Walk

▶Begin your walk at the hotel's front entrance on 15th Avenue.

▶Turn right on Yamhill and turn right. Walk three blocks north to the MAX Station on 18th Avenue.

▶Cross the street, using the traffic signals, into the entrance to the Jeld-Wen soccer stadium.

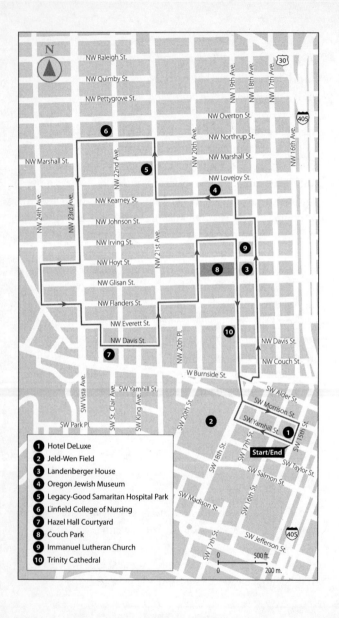

N

NW Raleigh St.
NW Quimby St.
NW Pettygrove St.
NW Overton St.
NW Northrup St.
NW Marshall St.
NW Marshall St.
NW Lovejoy St.
NW Kearney St.
NW Johnson St.
NW Irving St.
NW Hoyt St.
NW Glisan St.
NW Flanders St.
NW Everett St.
NW Davis St.
NW Davis St.
NW Couch St.
W Burnside St.
SW Vista Ave.
SW Yamhill St.
SW Park Pl.
SW St. Clair Ave.
SW King St.
SW Alder St.
SW Morrison St.
SW Yamhill St.
SW Taylor St.
SW Salmon St.
SW Madison St.
SW Jefferson St.

NW 24th Ave.
NW 23rd Ave.
NW 22nd Ave.
NW 21st Ave.
NW 20th Ave.
NW 20th Pl.
NW 19th Ave.
NW 18th Ave.
NW 17th Ave.
NW 16th Ave.
SW 20th St.
SW 18th St.
SW 17th St.
SW 16th St.
SW 17th St.

Start/End

30
405
405

1 Hotel DeLuxe
2 Jeld-Wen Field
3 Landenberger House
4 Oregon Jewish Museum
5 Legacy-Good Samaritan Hospital Park
6 Linfield College of Nursing
7 Hazel Hall Courtyard
8 Couch Park
9 Immanuel Lutheran Church
10 Trinity Cathedral

0   500 ft.
0   200 m.

▶Walk right to the six-foot-tall happy-face sculpture on the plaza at Morrison and 18th, installed when the seventy-year-old Civic Stadium became home to the Portland Timbers soccer team.

▶Cross Morrison and take the sidewalk alongside 19th Avenue down toward Burnside. You are on the left side of the triangular-shaped Firefighters Park. Cross 19th to the white limestone memorial fountain, dedicated to Captain David Campbell and all Portland firefighters who have died in the line of duty. Behind this is the largest bell in Portland, which once announced fires to all within hearing: "Hurry, Portland, it's time to serve your city." When new alert systems were implemented some sixty years ago, the bell was placed in storage. Now it has been resurrected and was placed here when the Firefighters Memorial was rededicated in 2000.

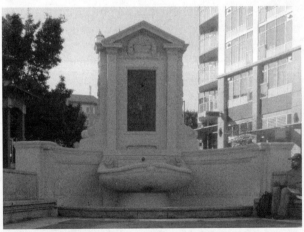

David Campbell memorial honors Portland firefighters.

Dick Lukins

▶Cross 18th at the foot of the Campbell fountain, and then cross Alder.

▶Cross Burnside at the traffic signal, and continue up the hill to Couch (pronounced "kooch") Street. Signs above the street names announce you're in the Alphabet District, on the western part of Captain John Couch's land claim.

CAPTAIN JOHN COUCH

This Alphabet (or Couch) District is the original land claim of John Couch, a sea captain from Newburyport, Massachusetts. Like many captains of the day, he had been in most major seaports of the world, and recognized a good port when he came up the Columbia River in 1840 and saw "The Clearing." This was a small stopping place nearby belonging to the Multnomah Indians, and used by travelers going upriver. Couch obtained a land claim in 1849, and chose to lay out his claim on true north, since he had spent his maritime career sailing by the North Star.

When surveyor Thomas Brown laid out the city in 1845, he used a compass, and his north-south streets conveniently paralleled the river. (He may not have realized that, in Portland, magnetic north deviates 21 degrees east from geographic or true north.) The mismatch between the streets north and south of Burnside creates several odd-shaped blocks, as well as a challenge to later traffic planners.

Captain Couch must have been a methodical man. He kept the existing system for the north-south avenues—1st, 2nd, and so forth—but chose to name his east-west streets with letters of the alphabet—A, B, C, etc. Later citizens replaced these with the names of noted Portlanders, but kept the alphabetical order.

The Roman Catholic Cathedral of Saint Mary of the Immaculate Conception is on the northeast corner of 18th and Couch. Built in 1925 and recently restored, this classic structure is graced with lovely bronze doors. This is still an active church, as evidenced by the large parking lot behind it on the other side of Davis.

▶Cross Davis, passing the parking lot. This was once the site of the Richard B. Knapp House. As you walk to Everett, you can see the remains of the original garden wall on the right side of the sidewalk.

▶Cross Everett at the traffic signal. At the northwest corner is the former First Church of Christ Scientist, built in the Beaux Arts style in 1909. Now it's the Northwest Neighborhood Cultural Center.

▶Continue north for two more blocks toward Glisan Street (pronounced "Gleason"). Just before you reach this street, you will pass the former Elliston Apartments, built in 1889. The building, now known as the Wickersham, is on the National Register of Historic Places. Note the whimsical bike rack along the street, shaped like one of the steaming teacups at the corner tea shop.

►Cross Glisan. C. A. Landenberger built the beautiful Queen Anne house on the northwest corner directly in front of you in 1896.

►Continue two more blocks to Irving Street. On the northeast are three well-kept Victorians, very similar, but each with distinctive architectural details.

►Cross Irving and continue to Johnson Street. Turn left onto Johnson. The Ayer-Shea House at number 1809 was built in 1892, and is considered one of this district's premier buildings.

►Cross 19th, then Johnson. Go one block to Kearney.

►Cross Kearney and turn left. Number 1953, the low, green building up the street on your right, is the Oregon Jewish Museum, containing a variety of displays about this aspect of Portland's history. Many Jewish immigrants came here from Russia in the early part of the twentieth century, when young men were conscripted into the czar's army and faced almost certain death.

►Proceed west three blocks, to 21st Avenue.

►Cross 21st Avenue and turn right onto Lovejoy. You will see the buildings of the Legacy Good Samaritan Hospital campus. The pleasant little park on the corner by the MAX line has tables and benches for sitting. Just inside the entrance are restrooms and a Healing Garden, open to the public.

▶Continue on 21st. Just before Marshall Street you'll pass the Anglican Church Cathedral of Saint Mark, a Romanesque church with a distinctive wheel window above the entrance.

▶Cross Marshall, and continue to Northrup Street. Cross Northrup and turn left. Continue west for a block and a half, crossing 22nd Avenue. The brick buildings on your right are part of the Linfield College–Good Samaritan School of Nursing. Founded in 1895, this was the first nursing school in Oregon, and is the Portland Branch of McMinnville's Linfield College.

▶Turn right into the small courtyard between the two buildings and look for the statue of Saint Francis surrounded by five large ravens. Then return to Northrup.

▶Continue west to 23rd Avenue. Turn left. Your nose will inform you that you are entering a popular eating and shopping area. On pleasant days, outdoor chairs and tables line the sidewalks, inviting you to sit, eat, and watch passersby. Walk south on either side of 23rd (or "Trendy-third"), past interesting shops and restaurants. Stop at the corner of Lovejoy Street. In front of the Nob Hill Bar & Grill on the southwest corner are three large metal pigs: Porky, Petunia, and Porklandia. Porklandia is the one with little piglets underneath. The artist, Joe Justice, lives in the neighborhood and visits them frequently.

▶Continue south along 23rd to the northeast corner of Irving, and admire Rupert Van Dazzle, the horse of many

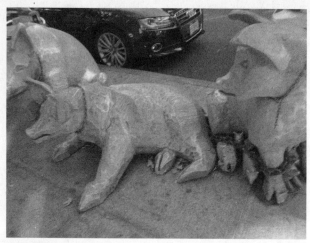
Porklandia is the mother sow in this group of pigs.

colors. The owner of the Dazzle shop brought him over from England when she originally opened the store, and he's been a colorful landmark ever since. He rides a skateboard into the shop at night and back out to the sidewalk every morning.

▶Continue one block to Hoyt. Turn right (west) on Hoyt and go up the hill one block to 24th Avenue.

▶Turn left here and proceed up the hill for two more blocks to Flanders Street, where 24th Avenue merges with Westover Road at the top of the hill. This area was originally too steep for building lots, but a hydraulic company brought in huge water flumes and sluiced unwanted earth down to the bottom of the hill. The dirt was used to fill in Guild Lake at Vaughn Street, once the site of the 1905 Lewis and

Clark Centennial Exposition. The company then terraced the hill and developed it as Westover Terraces, giving the streets aristocratic-sounding Virginia names.

▶Turn left on Flanders. The next three old homes you pass are also on the National Register of Historic Places. The Bates-Seller House, with its large porches, is a good example of the Queen Anne mixture of styles. Note the Ionic capitals on the columns on the first story and the Corinthian capitals on the second-story columns. East of the Bates-Seller House is the more-classical Charles F. Adams House. The next one to the east, the Trevett-Nunn House, displays a typical Colonial Revival symmetry.

▶You are now back on 23rd Avenue. Turn right and go one block south to Everett. Cross Everett, cross 23rd, and go east for one block to 22nd Place. Cross 22nd Place and turn right on the east side of the block. The plaque in front of number 106 tells you this was the home of Hazel Hall, a wheelchair-bound young seamstress who spent much of her life sewing for the fine ladies of the area. She saw life only through the diamond windows above the porch, but became one of Portland's most well-known poets. Today a prestigious Oregon poetry award carries her name. On the north side of the home is a small courtyard. Several of Hall's poems are inscribed on concrete tablets under a shady tree.

▶Go east through the center of the square and through the parking lot. Cross 22nd Avenue, and you will find yourself on Davis Street. Continue to 21st Avenue. You can see how this area is becoming increasingly desirable.

▸Turn left on 21st and go two blocks to Flanders. Cross 21st and walk toward 20th, passing several large old apartment houses with myriad architectural details. The first one is the 1907 Day Apartment Building. It is listed in the National Register, as is the George F. Heusner House on the corner of 20th and Flanders. Go around the corner to see its lovely entrance on 20th. Notice the graceful lines of the diamond-paned windows contrasting with the heavy stone foundation.

▸Go back to Flanders, cross 20th, and continue north. Cross Glisan carefully into Couch Park. To your left is the building of the former Couch School, now the Metropolitan Learning Center. Children from all over Portland attend this public K–12 school with its unique project-based curriculum. The remainder of the land given by Captain Couch has become this busy neighborhood park.

▸Go straight down the walkway in front of you to Hoyt Street. To your left, diagonally across the street at 2023 NW Hoyt, is the house built in the Richardsonian Romanesque style in 1892 for Dr. F. William Mackenzie. He was one of the founders of the University of Oregon Medical School, originally located nearby. The house is massive, and features a stone tower and windows recessed into rock walls. Note the cast-iron embellishments, such as a sun decorating the stone chimney, and the antlered stag—part of the Mackenzie family crest—peering down from an upper window. Scotch thistles are carved in the woodwork. It is now known as the William Temple House, a counseling center operated by the Episcopal Diocese of Oregon.

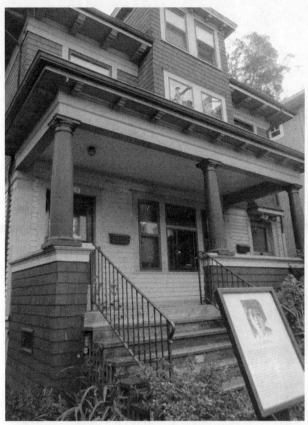

Crippled by polio, seamstress Hazel Hall stitched her own life, writing poetry behind the upstairs window.

▶Continue north to Irving and turn right. Across 20th is the Immanuel Lutheran Church, founded in 1879 as a Swedish Lutheran church, and built in 1906. It still holds a Christmas Day service in Swedish.

▸Turn right on 19th and continue back to Hoyt. Cross and walk to Glisan along the edge of Couch Park. Stop at the corner of Glisan to get a good view of Temple Beth Israel and its grounds, built where Captain Couch's brother-in-law, George Flanders, once lived. Only the low stone wall around the property remains. Admire the Carpenter Gothic–style house on the east side of 19th before crossing Glisan at the light.

▸You can see the tower of Trinity Cathedral as you continue up the slight hill on your way to cross Everett. The bright red entrance doors of this Episcopal cathedral catch the eye. The Rosales pipe organ here, described as "bright, thundering, [and] majestic," has 4,194 pipes, and is considered one of the premier organs in the United States. Music lovers visit the cathedral to admire the organ; others come to admire the needlepoint kneelers. Designed and made by parishioners, each depicts a different Oregon flower.

▸Continue south on 19th. The cathedral gardens on your right were once used by the marching band of the private Bishop Scott School.

▸Go down the modest hill to Burnside Street. Cross Burnside at the traffic signal and continue up past Firefighters Park to the junction of 19th and 18th. Cross, then turn left on Morrison. Go east three blocks, to 15th. Cross Morrison to the entrance.

Walk 6: Goose Hollow, Kings Hill, and the West End

📷 ✕ 🛒 🏢

General location: Downtown Portland

Special attractions: The Goose Hollow Inn, a city view from Vista Bridge, historic mansions, and a major league soccer stadium that pays homage to its history

Difficulty: Moderate

Distance: 3 miles

Estimated time: 1.5 hours

Services: Restaurants, restrooms, and water

Restrictions: This walk is not suitable for wheelchairs. Narrow sidewalks, few curb cuts, and uphill sections also make it difficult for strollers.

For more information: Contact the Portland Oregon Visitors Association.

Getting started: The walk starts at the Ace Hotel on Stark Street, between 10th and 11th Avenues. To reach the hotel from I-5 northbound, take the exit to I-405, and then take the Salmon Street exit. From I-5 southbound, take exit 302B to I-405, then the Couch-Burnside exit. Metered parking is available on the street. A "Smart Park" garage is under the 9th and Stark Street entrance to O'Bryant Park.

Public transportation: The N-S Portland streetcar stops at 11th and Alder, SB, 10th and Alder NB. The MAX light-rail system transit center is at Pioneer Place, between 5th and 6th Avenues.

Overview: Early Portland included stump-filled land, good soil, and gulches filled with water runoff from the Tualatin Hills. These attracted a wide variety of workers, immigrants from many lands, and a wealthy merchant class that grew rich along with the city. This walk takes you from the once-depressed commercial area, newly attractive to today's young entrepreneurs, to a working-class area known for its tannery and Chinese gardens, to the well-kept mansions overlooking the once-busy city. On the way you will also pass by one of Portland's oldest sports fields, newly renovated into a major league soccer stadium.

The Walk

▶Start at the Ace Hotel, 1022 SW Stark Street. This hotel reflects what *The Oregonian* describes as the "funky urban vibe of the West End." Even the lobby is low-key, with comfy couches and a welcoming coffee fragrance. Begin your walk at the front entrance on Stark Street.

▶Walk east to SW 10th Avenue. Turn right and walk to Washington Street, passing the Portland Institute for Contemporary Art in the bright-colored building on your right. The Pittock Block Building across the street was the site of Henry Pittock's former mansion, before he moved up to Pittock's Mansion (now a city park), sitting high atop the West Hills, northwest of Burnside. This large structure was built in 1912 by the recently expanding electric company.

▶Turn right on Washington. A variety of restaurants and interesting, small owner–run shops—vintage clothing,

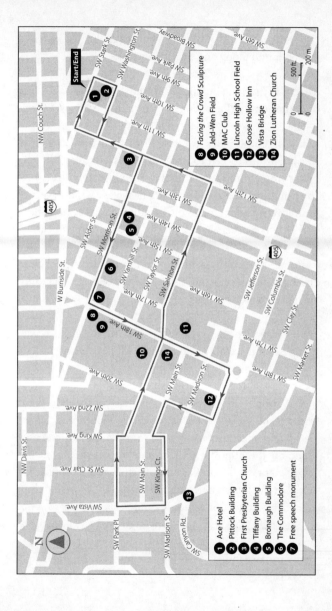

Start/End

Legend (right box):

8 *Facing the Crowd* Sculpture
9 Jeld-Wen Field
10 MAC Club
11 Lincoln High School Field
12 Goose Hollow Inn
13 Vista Bridge
14 Zion Lutheran Church

Legend (bottom box):

1 Ace Hotel
2 Pittock Building
3 First Presbyterian Church
4 Tiffany Building
5 Bronaugh Building
6 The Commodore
7 Free speech monument

Scale: 0 — 500 ft; 0 — 200 m.

Street labels:
NW Couch St., SW Stark St., SW Washington St., SW Park Ave, SW 9th Ave, SW 10th Ave, SW 11th Ave, SW Broadway, SW 6th Ave, W Burnside St., SW Alder St., SW Morrison St., SW Yamhill St., SW Taylor St., SW Salmon St., SW 13th Ave, SW 14th Ave, SW 15th Ave, SW 16th Ave, SW 17th Ave, SW 18th Ave, SW Jefferson St., SW Columbia St., SW Clay St., SW Market St., SW 12th Ave, SW Main St., SW Madison St., SW Kings Ct., SW 20th Ave, SW 22nd Ave, SW King Ave, SW St. Clair Ave, SW Vista Ave, SW Park Pl., NW Davis St., SW Canyon Rd., 405

children's toys, and a milliner who makes hats to order—can be found along and near this street.

▸Cross 11th to the building with the clock tower. This was once the home of Pittock's newspaper, the *Portland Telegram*.

▸Continue one block west to 12th, then turn and cross Washington. Proceed to Alder and cross. Cross 12th. You are in front of the First Presbyterian Church with its historic architecture and Povey stained-glass windows. Pass their lovely gardens, open during lunch hours so neighbors and nearby workers have a pleasant place to sit and eat.

▸Go one block to Morrison Street, and turn right. Note the signs that detail the history of the church, including the Povey windows.

▸Proceed east on Morrison. Cross 13th and the freeway overpass. You are now in the Goose Hollow District.

▸Cross 14th and then Morrison by the Tiffany Building at the corner. The lovely doors invite you to open them and step inside to the gracious vintage lobby. You can see period elegance in every detail, from the romantic Venice scene on the opposite wall, to the tile on the floor. The large seal of the Grand Circle of Neighbors of Woodcraft is inlaid in the center, under a round table. Now the building is used as a venue for weddings and gala events.

The next building, the Bronaugh at 1434 Morrison, was built in 1905. It is the oldest-surviving apartment house in Portland, and has fascinating architectural details on its facade.

▶Cross 15th. On your left is the classic-looking Scottish Rite Center. This was built in 1902, and is now another popular event venue. Across the street is the modern Artists Repertory Theatre, which offers many contemporary plays.

▶Cross 16th. The Commodore, the gold building across the street with the Egyptian style trim, was built in 1927, and is one of Portland's few authentic Art Deco apartment buildings.

▶Continue to 17th and cross to the small corner plaza at the MAX train stop. (Watch out for the crossing trains.)

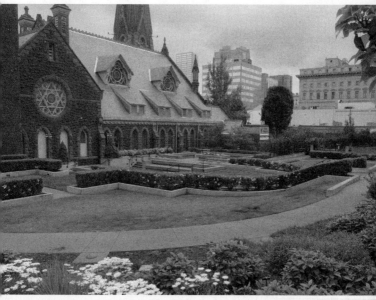

Povey stained-glass windows grace Historic First Presbyterian Church. *Dick Lukins*

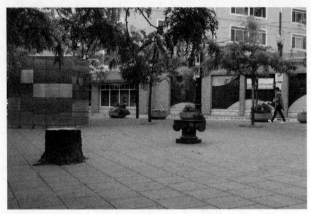

A stump awaits a stump speech at this MAX station. *Dick Lukins*

Note the quotations engraved on the large aluminum lockers in the center, a monument to the right of free speech. A concrete stump, a soapbox, and a capital of a Roman column beg for a speaker of the day, and forum-style benches await an audience.

▶Cross 18th to the corner of the Jeld-Wen Stadium (originally Multnomah Stadium and Civic Stadium), where a six-foot-high happy face greets you. Sculptor Michael Stutz created *Facing the Crowd* to remind us about the importance of maintaining humor in the midst of a chaotic urban world. A duplicate is at the 20th Avenue entrance.

▶Take the walkway to your left to the gate in front of the Timbers Store. If it is open, enter and go to the south wall of the building. In a Portland Timbers soccer game, "Timber Joey" saws off a log slab after the team scores a goal.

That ceremony inspired sculptor Ron Baron to use a slab to honor the field's past. Embedded within the tree rings are many artifacts representing the field's long history: antlers, vegetables, a fish, Chinese figures, all sorts of sports memorabilia, and even little cat figures for the feral cats that have lived beneath the stadium for decades.

▶Take a look at the recently remodeled stadium from the plaza. Legend has it that the large tannery vats are still buried under the field. As the West Hills area was being developed, all the debris was dumped into the gullies and ravines to level out this plain. On the south side you can see the Multnomah Athletic Club (MAC) building.

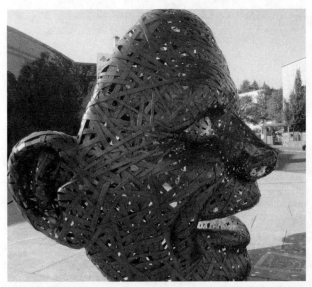

Facing the Crowd at Jeld-Wen Stadium keeps its sense of humor.

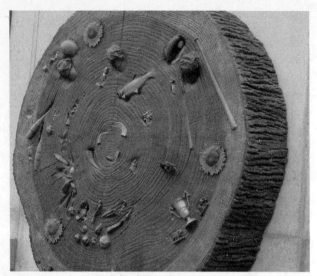

Reminders of area history are embedded in the slab. *Dick Lukins*

▶Exit through the gates and turn south. Note the pavement block telling about the ski jump that took place here back in 1951. The iron fencing along the stadium lets you see what's going on inside.

▶If the next set of gates is open, go in to see large panels showing the history of Goose Hollow. They can also be viewed from outside, through the fence. One panel shows the route of Tanner Creek as it meandered through the gulches to Couch Lake, now part of the Pearl District near Union Station. Today it runs through huge underground pipes, surfacing at Tanner Springs Park, also in the Pearl.

GOOSE HOLLOW HISTORY

Tanner Creek was named for the tannery on its banks that Daniel Lownsdale opened in 1845. This creek still flows through massive pipes under the area, surfacing at Tanner Creek Park in the Pearl District. It was a good site, with access to flowing water and hickory trees nearby. (The latter was important, as the rawhides were soaked for six months in a hickory-bark mixture.) It was also a smelly trade, best done far away from residential areas. The tannery was the only one west of the Rockies.

Later, Lownsdale turned his attention to building the Great Plank Road. From the Tualatin Valley to the west, the Plank Road followed present-day Canyon Road and the Sunset Highway 26 over the West Hills. As it entered Portland through Goose Hollow, it connected with SW Market Street Drive on the southern slope above the hollow. Amos King bought the tannery land and rented it to Chinese farmers, who found that the rich soil washed down from the hills made for productive vegetable gardens.

More immigrants flowed into this area, mainly Irish and Germans. The name originated from the Oregonian report of "A War about Geese." These birds roamed freely throughout the gulch (hollow), demolished gardens, and kept neighbors awake at night. When a police officer responded to the many complaints, a dozen women owners drove him off, and the area became known as the hollow where women squabbled about geese.

In 1967, Bud Clark—who later became one of Portland's most colorful mayors—chose the formerly disparaging name of Goose Hollow for his newly purchased tavern. It became well-known, as did its owner, when Bud Clark posed for the "Expose Yourself to Art" poster. The Goose Hollow name is now flaunted with pride, and banners adorn many local homes and shops.

The advent of the streetcar on "B" Street (Burnside) made it possible for the wealthy to build houses up on the heights of Amos King's Hill. These homes afforded great views and were separated from the workingmen's cottages below. (The streetcar company built houses on the hill for its conductors.) Much of the sluiced-off soil from mansion construction filled the creeks and hollows below. Where once you would have had to pick your way through rivulets, gulches, and mud, walking through the now-flat area is easy.

In 1892 the Multnomah Amateur Athletic Club, now known as the MAC, leased some Chinese garden land for an athletic field. A clubhouse and grandstand followed, and were used for many sporting events. After a fire, the new clubhouse was built on Salmon Street. Over the years, the field took over the former produce farms, and Multnomah Field became Multnomah Stadium, and later still, Civic Stadium. Celebrities like Elvis Presley and Marilyn Monroe appeared here.

▶After you are through reading the history panels, take the crosswalk to the traffic signal and the MAX platform in the center of 18th Avenue. Admire the statue of the bronze goose on the platform, and note the river-shaped paving with more reminders of Goose Hollow history. Then take the south crosswalk at Salmon to the east side of 18th.

▶Turn right, crossing Salmon. The Lincoln High School athletic field is on your left, somewhat hidden by the large fence. The fence has become an art wall, with tiles, cut-outs, and creative pictures providing a glimpse of high school life.

▶Continue walking south, looking for more inscribed paving blocks underfoot. Another student art project, these inscriptions commemorate Goose Hollow history. The first one is a sketch of Bart Simpson by his creator, Matt Groening, a 1972 graduate of Lincoln High. Others have brief histories of the first teacher, the Chinese gardens, and even the names of Goose Hollow pets. Unfortunately, many weren't scratched in deeply enough and are becoming difficult to read.

▶Stop at the Jefferson Street traffic signal. This, along with Market Street (now a block east of here), was the site of the Great Plank Road. It gave access from the Tualatin Valley to the west, allowing commercial quantities of farm products to reach Portland for consumption and distribution—another factor in its evolution as a commercial center.

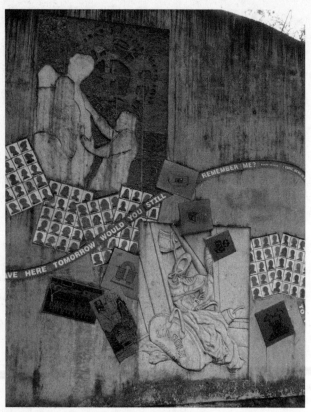

Art graces the Lincoln High School athletic field fence.

Dick Lukins

▶Turn right and cross 18th, walking west along Jefferson. Another MAX station is on your left. Stay on this north side, cross 19th, and you are at the Goose Hollow Inn. This site was once a beer garden for German immigrants using their gymnastics club—the Turn-Verein-Gymnasium up the street.

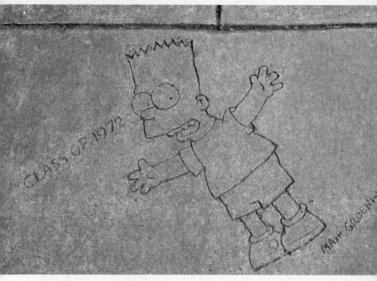

This drawing of Bart Simpson is by Matt Groening, a Lincoln High School alum. *Dick Lukins*

▶Continue straight to 20th Avenue. Before you cross and turn right, look for the manhole in the street. If you go to it and listen, and the traffic is quiet, you can hear the burble of Tanner Creek down below, still draining the West Hills. Another manhole cover at the west end of the MAX station is also a good listening spot.

▶Continue across 20th Avenue and turn right. Walk two blocks to Main. Turn left on Main Street and go up the hill to King Street. Turn left for half a block on King Street, and then turn right onto King's Court. You are now in the King's Hill neighborhood, walking past lovely historic homes.

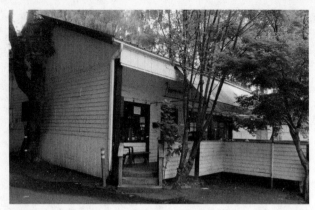

The owner of Goose Hollow Inn became a Portland mayor and brought fame to the area.

▸Ascend the two blocks on this charming small street, passing the Portland Garden Club as you reach Vista Avenue.

▸Turn left to cross the 1926 Vista Bridge, a famous landmark with marvelous views as it arches over Jefferson Street. Small niches at each end contain benches, part of the original design.

▸Retrace your steps across the bridge and continue north on this side to Park Place. Look west up the hill to see the formal entrance to Washington Park, marked by a brick retaining wall.

▸Turn right (east) on Park Place. Descend, crossing St. Clair to King Street. Turn right to Salmon Street.

▸Cross King and descend on the left side of Salmon, passing the walled sunken garden next to the redbrick Town

Club. Cross 21st and 20th. The Chinese produce farms were located where the MAC Club now stands. Go to 18th.

▶Across on the south side of Salmon, Zion Lutheran Church nestles unobtrusively into the surroundings. Designed by Pietro Belluschi, its use of light and wood enhances and complements the congregation's worship. Zion Lutheran is listed as one of Portland's historic buildings.

▶Go to 18th. Cross Salmon and 18th to Lincoln Field. The field and high school buildings are on your right.

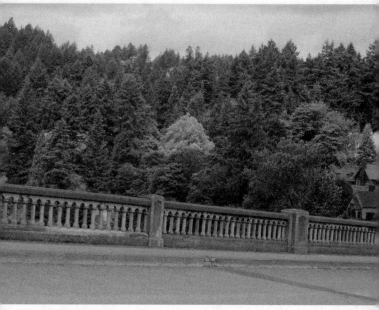

Vista Bridge arches gracefully over Jefferson Street.
Dick Lukins

▸Proceed east on Salmon, crossing 14th to the overpass to 13th Avenue. Cross 13th and continue east on Salmon to 12th.

▸Turn left on 12th, crossing Salmon, and go six blocks north to Stark Street.

▸Turn right, cross 11th, and you will find yourself passing by the Stumptown Coffee Roasters shop as you return to your starting place at the Ace Hotel.

FOREST PARK (WEST)

Walk 7: Audubon Bird Sanctuary

General location: Forest Park on the northwest side of Portland

Special attractions: A natural environment, home to birds and other wildlife

Difficulty: Moderate; dirt and gravel paths wind up and down slopes

Distance: 1 mile

Estimated time: 1 hour

Services: Water, restrooms, nature store with an emphasis on birds and wildlife habitat

Restrictions: Trails are open dawn to dusk. The Audubon House Interpretive Center and Nature Store are open from 10 a.m. to 6 p.m. daily, except on Sunday, when they close at 5 p.m. No dogs, smoking, bicycling, or littering permitted on the trail.

For more information: Contact the Portland Audubon Society and Nature Store, 5151 Northwest Cornell Road Portland, OR 97210; (503) 292-9453; audubonportland .org.

Getting started: From I-5 northbound, exit onto I-405 northbound. Take this to the Everett Street exit. Proceed two blocks to Glisan Street. Turn left onto Glisan. Continue to NW 21st, go to Lovejoy Street, and turn left (west).

From I-5 southbound, exit onto I-405 southbound. Take this to the Glisan Street exit. At the first traffic light (on Glisan, a one-way street) continue straight ahead for two blocks to Everett, turn left, left again for two blocks, and left again onto Glisan. Continue to NW 21st, go to Lovejoy Street, and turn left (west). Proceed past 25th Avenue where Lovejoy becomes Cornell Road. Continue west about 1.5 miles through two tunnels to Audubon House, 5151 NW Cornell, on the right side of the road.

Public transportation: None

Overview: The Portland Audubon Society operates Audubon House, an interpretive center with exhibits of birds and wildlife. They also run a wildlife rehabilitation center specializing in birds. The excellent nature store features gifts, books, and aids for identifying the birds, wildlife, and plants you may see along the trail. A trail map shows three loop walks that begin at the store. The society offers many different birding events, nature classes, and guided tours, so call for information on times and dates.

The Walk

▶Start your walk at the Portland Audubon House and Nature Store. Enjoy the exhibits inside and find out about the activities that may be happening during your visit. Pick up a trail map. There are several trails to choose from; the one described here is the Pittock Sanctuary Nature Trail.

▶Walk to the east end of the covered walkway. The trail begins here.

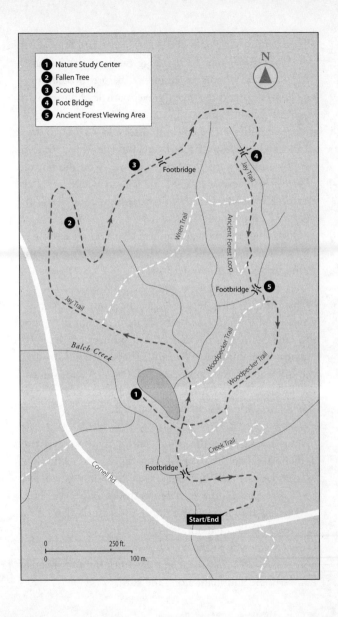

N

1 Nature Study Center
2 Fallen Tree
3 Scout Bench
4 Foot Bridge
5 Ancient Forest Viewing Area

3 Footbridge

4 Jay Trail

2

Wren Trail

Ancient Forest Loop

Footbridge 5

Jay Trail

Balch Creek

Woodpecker Trail

Woodpecker Trail

1

Creek Trail

Cornell Rd

Footbridge

Start/End

0   250 ft.
0   100 m.

▶Turn left onto the path at the end of the building and go down the stone steps to the large outdoor animal cages. Stop and see who is in residence before descending a wooden ramp and the steep gravel path leading to Balch Creek. This rain-fed stream was named for one of Oregon's pioneer families with a colorful history. It is home to some landlocked native cutthroat trout, and the American Dipper, an unusual bird that swims or walks on the bottom of streams in search of food. Be careful where you step: the creek is fragile, subject to erosion that could harm the plants or animals in it.

Birds singing overhead confirm that you are entering a birder's paradise. Small signs identify some of the plants found in this mixed-conifer forest.

▶Cross the Balch Creek Bridge and continue past the Creek Trail toward the pond, named in honor of Samantha Jane Seaman. An Oregon Trail pioneer of 1852, she "cared for the birds for 75 years." Thick growth surrounds the still water. If you look carefully, you may spot some of the resident turtles, frogs, newts, and giant salamanders. The Nature Study Shelter is at your left.

▶After investigating the pond, return to the gravel trail and continue on the Jay Trail. Hawthorns and wildflowers border the path, flowering in season. Stay on the path as it bends left, passing the entrance to the Woodpecker Trail.

The Jay Trail follows the north and east borders of the sanctuary. Trillium abounds in the spring, and vine maple is easy to identify in the fall since it is one of the few Oregon native trees that turns red. Sword ferns and maidenhair ferns are abundant along the path.

▶Continue up the Jay Trail, ignoring side trails. Pass by the entrance to the Wren Trail. Sword ferns and Oregon grape cover the bank on your right. You can hear the city traffic as you go uphill from Balch Creek. The sound fades away as you continue around to the right. Go up a few steps on the trail as you move away from the road. You will notice many trees—fallen and standing—that act as nurse logs for new plants.

▶Continue going up a ridge, crossing under the trunk of a fallen tree supported by living ones.

▶Continue along the narrow and twisting Jay Trail to an Eagle Scout bench. Sitting on it, you can almost believe you are in a wilderness instead of a busy city. If you sit long enough, and quietly enough, you may see some pileated woodpeckers (the ones that resemble Woody the Woodpecker, with their red crowns).

▶Leave the bench and continue on the path. Cross a footbridge. As the path starts down, you can see buildings beyond the sanctuary boundary on the other side of a shallow ravine.

▶Cross a second footbridge. You are entering an old-growth area. Pass the intersection with the Wren Trail, and continue on the Jay Trail. On your right you will see a small clearing, centered by a giant Douglas fir. A viewing platform with benches surrounds the tree that is riddled with holes all the way to the top. The rectangular holes are made by pileated woodpeckers, drilling for insects. The paths under the tall firs seem small and almost hidden, making you feel like one of the early explorers. Decaying stumps and snags act as nurse logs for many new plants.

►Cross the footbridge and stay on the Jay Trail until it intersects with the Woodpecker Trail. Turn left. Ignore side trails as you return to the pond and the Nature Study Shelter. This pavilion provides a pleasant place to rest and have a snack, while looking for the turtles relaxing on floating logs.

►Then take the path back up to your starting point at Audubon House.

Walk 8: Washington Park North

General location: 1 mile west of downtown Portland

Special attractions: Playgrounds, the International Rose Test Garden, tennis courts, and the Oregon Holocaust Memorial; there is access to the Japanese Gardens and a train during the summer that takes you to the nearby Washington Park Zoo.

Difficulty: Moderate. This park is made up of a series of terraces climbing up a steep slope. You will be climbing steps and taking one gravel trail, though most of it is on paved roads.

Distance: 2 miles

Estimated time: 1 hour

Services: Restrooms and water are available by the Garden Store and at the Oregon Holocaust Memorial.

Restrictions: Washington Park and the International Rose Test Garden are open daily during daylight hours. The garden shop and the zoo train are not open in winter.

For more information: Contact the Portland Oregon Visitors Association, 701 Southwest 6th Avenue, Portland, OR 97204; (503) 275-8355; travelportland.com; or Portland Parks and Recreation, 1120 SW 5th Avenue #1302, Portland, OR 97204; (503) 823-PLAY (7529); portlandonline.com/park.

Getting started: From I-405 (northbound), take the Salmon Street exit; proceed until you take a left onto Burnside. From I-405 (southbound), take the Burnside exit and proceed to a right onto Burnside. From either

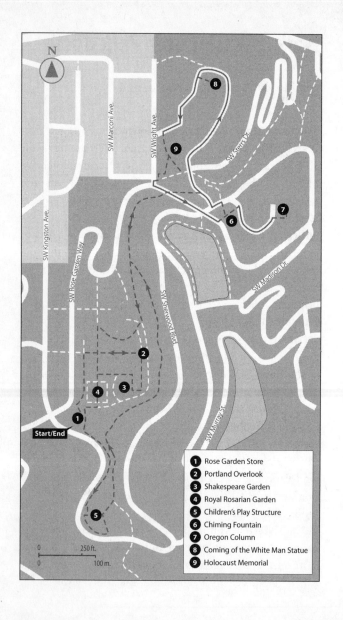

N

SW Marconi Ave.

SW Wright Ave.

SW Kingston Ave.

SW Sherds Dr.

SW Rose Garden Way

SW Madison Dr.

SW Sherwood Blvd

SW Murray St.

Start/End

1 Rose Garden Store
2 Portland Overlook
3 Shakespeare Garden
4 Royal Rosarian Garden
5 Children's Play Structure
6 Chiming Fountain
7 Oregon Column
8 Coming of the White Man Statue
9 Holocaust Memorial

0   250 ft.
0   100 m.

direction, take Burnside west to Tichner, the fourth signal past 23rd Street. Turn left on Tichnor. At the top of the hill, turn right on Kingston. The Rose Garden Store is at the second stop sign, at the end of the tennis courts. Park by the tennis courts or in the store parking lot. There are year round restrooms and a picnic area here.

Public transportation: TriMet Bus 63 (Washington Park) stops at the International Rose Test Garden, Japanese Gardens, and the Washington Park Zoo. The Washington Park and Zoo Railway travels between the rose gardens and Washington Park Zoo, where there is a MAX light-rail station.

Overview: This 332-acre park offers sweeping panoramic views, play and picnic areas, tennis courts, a zoo, and an amphitheater for outdoor concerts. It is one of Portland's oldest and best-loved parks. Former German sailor Charles Meyers, the first park keeper, relied on his memories of European parks as he developed what was then called City Park. Former seaman Richard Knight, a Portland pharmacist, had begun purchasing the animals collected by his old shipmates during their travels. When his acquisitions outgrew his exhibition space, he donated the animals to the city for a zoo. Meyers added the role of zookeeper to his duties. He dug the world's first sunken pit to house the zoo's bears.

John Olmsted, of the famous firm of landscape architects, was designing parks for Seattle in 1903. During a visit to Portland, he made several suggestions for park improvements, including changing City Park's name to Washington Park.

The Walk

►Start this walk at the large map of the park outside the Rose Garden Store. Turn to your right and continue straight north on the sidewalk along the road with parking. (Note: A handicapped-accessible walkway into the Rose Garden descends from the Garden Store's restrooms.)

►At the second opening in the stone wall, take the steps to your right that lead to the information kiosk. Here you can see maps showing the park's layout of the many roses in the International Rose Test Garden.

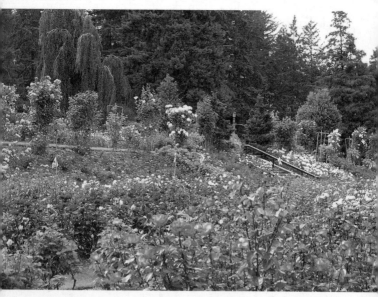

International Rose Test Garden contains more than 520 varieties of roses. *Portland Parks & Recreation, Portland, OR*

▶Pass the kiosk, continue on the walkway, and enjoy views of the city as you descend the steps and terraces among formal flower beds. These are test beds for those roses to be selected as "All-American." They contain more than 520 varieties of roses of almost every imaginable hue—reds, lavenders, oranges, and whites. They come from all over the world.

▶Continue to the overlook at the end of this garden walkway, where winning selections are displayed. On a square in the center of the path is a bronze tile with the name of the current Rose Festival Queen. The overlook's view of snow-crowned Mount Hood shows up on many Portland posters and postcards.

▶Turn back to the walkway, turning south along the Queen's Walk. All past queens have their names and years inscribed on bronze tiles laid among the bricks.

▶Continue into the Shakespeare Garden. Turn right at the center walk. Plants mentioned in Shakespeare's plays fill the boxwood-bordered flower beds. This garden was planned as a counterpoint to the riotous colors of the roses.

▶Go to the brick alcove at the far end of the garden. A plaque displays Shakespeare's own quotation, "Of all the flowers methinks a rose is best."

▶Turn right to the path exiting the garden. Proceed north to the next main walkway.

▶Turn left and go up the steps under the rose trellises. The Gold Medal Test Gardens to your left contain roses especially adapted to the Northwest climate. After viewing these beds, continue up to the next terrace and the stainless-steel pillars of the Frank Beach Memorial Fountain. Lee Kelly designed this in honor of the man who first called Portland the "City of Roses." Children love playing on the fountain's stepping-stones.

▶Walk south at the fountain and enter the Royal Rosarian Garden, named for the civic leaders who sponsor Portland's annual Rose Festival. It is planted with their namesake roses. The Prime Minister's Walk goes around the perimeter, and you can see the names of Rosarians inscribed on the tiles along the path.

▶Leave by the Bill Bane bronze statue of a Royal Rosarian tipping his hat to you, and turn right on the road back to the Garden Store. Turn left at the store and exit on SW Sherwood Boulevard.

▶Turn south and stay left as you start down the hill. You will see and pass a flight of steps on the right side of the road. These lead up to the Washington Park and Zoo Railway Depot. This April–September railway carries passengers on a 35-minute, 4-mile round-trip to the Washington Park Zoo. This is the last official railroad in the United States to offer continual mail service. Letters deposited on the railway receive a special hand cancellation. There is a small fee to ride the train, and you must also pay for admission to the zoo. Contact the Washington Park Zoo for information on rates and schedules.

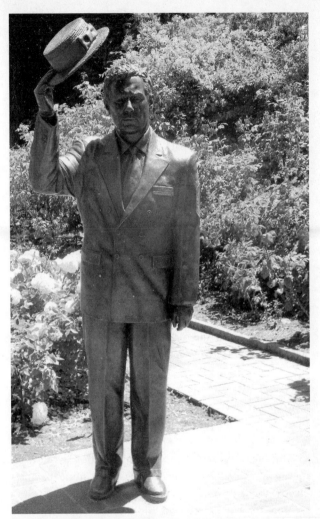

The Royal Rosarians are Portland's official greeters and goodwill ambassadors. *Dick Lukins*

▶Continue walking south on the left side of Sherwood Boulevard until you reach the children's play area. Large colorful structures invite children to stretch their muscles as well as their imagination.

▶Turn left between topiary llamas to enter the playground. Note the bronze map in Braille on the pedestal to your left. Turn right on the path toward the sandbox centered by a baby elephant statue, then take the path on your left toward the large play structure. Go underneath the play bridge on the left side of the circular slide.

▶Turn to your right toward the cement plinth marking a nature trail. This gravel path is a popular running path, part of the Multnomah Athletic Club trail system. You will see occasional MAC signs throughout this area of the park.

▶Continue on the trail for a half-mile past a little overlook. A service road is above you on the left. Below you to the right are Sherwood Road and a large reservoir.

▶Turn right when you connect with the service road. Continue to the white posts marking its end. Turn right.

▶Continue east down the road to its junction with Washington Way. Wrought-iron railings and stone parapets enclose the large reservoir on your right.

Note the large grassy knoll in front of you. Cross the road to the cast-iron fountain at the base. This is the 1891 Chiming Fountain, Swiss immigrant John Staehli's copy of a Renaissance fountain. Originally, a statue of a small boy stood on top of the fountain, but it was destroyed when water left in the fountain froze one winter.

▸Take the path to the left of the fountain. Go to the bronze statue of the Native American woman, Sacagawea, who served as translator and guide to explorers Lewis and Clark. She stands on a large rock, facing west, with her infant son on her back. Installed for the Lewis and Clark Centennial Exposition of 1905, this is the first public statue of a woman ever erected in the United States. Paid for by donations from women all over the country, suffragists Susan B. Anthony and Abigail Scott Duniway presided at its installation.

▸Turn right at Sacagawea. Go up the path between a pic-nic area and a children's play area. Continue to the Oregon Column on top of the knoll commemorating Meriwether Lewis and William Clark, the first official US explorers of the Oregon Country. President Theodore Roosevelt laid the foundation stone in 1903. Seals of Oregon, Idaho, Montana, and Washington—all part of the original Ore-gon Country—are displayed on the base's four sides.

▸Go around to the east side of the column to see how high you are above the downtown area. The steps in front of you go down to a brick wall crowned with flowers, Wash-ington Park's formal entrance on SW Park Place. The street descends down a steep slope into the city. It makes you realize how important the Chiming Fountain must have been to horses pulling carriages full of visitors up this hill.

▸Go back around the column and return to the cast-iron fountain.

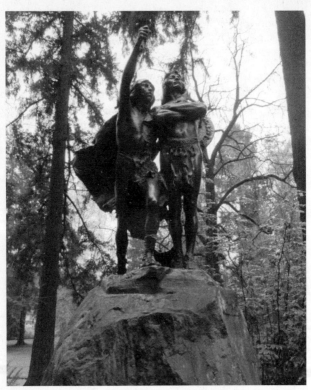

In *The Coming of the White Man,* the older man supposedly represents Chief Multnomah.

▶Cross to the road directly opposite the fountain, going through two white posts. Continue up through another set of posts, and you will be on a one-way road, Washington Way. You will be walking facing the traffic.

▶Continue on Washington Way up the hill, passing the entrance to Stearns Road. On the hillside below on the right, just past the lawn area, is the Cloud Forest rhododendron garden. This hillside was formerly overrun with invasive species. Through concerted efforts by the park and volunteer groups, the area was reclaimed, and a rhododendron garden has been established. This garden contains many different species, including several big-leaf varieties, a mix of interesting herbaceous perennials, and native companion plants that create a multilayered rhododendron woodland.

At the top of the hill is a small parking pullout. Another bronze sculpture, entitled *The Coming of the White Man,* is on the knoll.

The statue portrays a young Native American brave showing an elder some explorers coming down the Willamette River. The family of former Portland mayor David Thompson asked sculptor Herman McNeil to create this gift to the city in 1904. The sculptor supposedly modeled the older man after Chief Multnomah, who once lived near "The Clearing" on the Willamette River, where Portland was founded.

▶Continue on around Washington Way and turn left at a crosswalk into the Oregon Holocaust Memorial. Note the cast-iron objects scattered across the central square, a bleak reminder of the thousands of people who gathered in similar squares before leaving for the concentration camps.

▶Cross the square. Inlaid granite bars like railroad tracks mark the path as you journey to the large granite wall, where ashes of victims from each camp are buried. The facing side gives a history of the Holocaust, and inlaid blocks display quotations from Holocaust survivors. The polished granite on the reverse side gives the names of many Portlanders' relatives who perished in the camps.

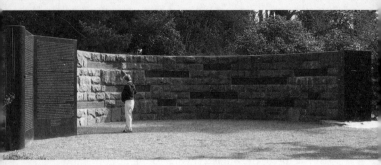

Soil and ash from six Holocaust killing camps are buried beneath the wall. *Portland Parks & Recreation, Portland, OR*

▸Return to the bench at the rear of the square, and exit on the west side of the brick restroom building. Cross the road at the pedestrian crossing to the service road ahead of you, marked by two white iron posts. (This is the same road you traveled earlier before exiting the Nature Trail.) Continue down this service road, past the entrance to the Nature Trail, until you come to a walkway on your right.

▸Turn right and take the path between two iron posts. Note the beautiful large, grassy amphitheater on your right. This is a popular venue for summer concerts, and the large arborvitae screen provides a perfect backdrop for summer plays. The Rose Gardens are on your left.

▸Continue up this walkway until you reach a T-junction.
    Turn left, and go south past the Frank Beach Memorial Fountain, and follow the walkway up to the Rose Garden Store. Tables and chairs here provide a welcome resting area, and the small store is packed with unique rose-related items to remind you of this delightful park.

At the map near the Rose Garden Store, notice the sign to the Japanese Gardens. These are not connected to the Rose Gardens, and have their own entrance fee. They are considered the most beautiful and authentic landscape of this type outside Japan, with five types of gardens that are lovely in each season of the year. Add this to your Rose Garden experience, or return on a separate visit. Maps and information are available at the entrance gate.

Walk 9: Washington Park South

🔲 👫 🏢 🍃 ♿

General location: West of downtown Portland

Special attractions: The Vietnam Memorial, the Hoyt Arboretum, the Children's Museum, the World Forestry Center, and the Portland Zoo

Difficulty: Easy walk on paved trails, with some uphill sections

Distance: About 2.5 miles

Estimated time: 2 hours

Services: Restrooms and water at the MAX station, and the Hoyt Center at the turnaround point on the trail

Restrictions: The park itself is open during daylight hours. The Children's Museum, the World Forestry Center, and the Portland Zoo have admission fees. Call the individual attractions for information on hours, days, and required fees.

For more information:

Portland Visitor Information Center, 701 SW 6th Avenue at Morrison Street, Portland, OR 97204; (503) 275-8355 or (800) 962-3700; travelportland.com.

Portland Parks and Recreation, 1120 SW 5th Avenue #1302, Portland, OR 97204; (503) 823-PLAY (7529); portlandonline.com/park.

Portland Zoo, 4001 SW Canyon Road, Portland, OR 97221; (503) 226-1561; oregonzoo.org.

Portland Children's Museum, 4015 Southwest Canyon Road, Portland, OR 97221; (503) 223-6500; portlandcm.org.

World Forestry Center, 4033 SW Canyon Road, Portland, OR 97221; (503) 228-1367; worldforestry.org.

Getting started: Take US 26 westbound. Then take the exit marked "Zoo-Forestry Center" and follow the road to the parking lot of the Zoo-Forestry Center at the MAX light-rail station.

South to Portland on I-5: Follow the signs for Beaverton and get on US 26 West. Go through the tunnel and up a gradual hill, then look for the Zoo-Forestry Center signs and exit 72. It's the first one you'll see on US 26.

North to Portland on I-5: Take exit 299B for Beaverton, which is just before you get downtown. This puts you on I-405. Take exit 1D to US 26 West. Go through the tunnel and up a gradual hill, then look for the Zoo-Forestry Center signs and exit 72. It's the first one you'll see on US 26.

West to Portland on I-84: Follow the signs for Beaverton and US 26 West.(See directions above.)

From Downtown Portland: Drive south on Broadway (or any of the numbered avenues) and turn west onto Clay Street. This street takes you right to US 26 West. Then take the first exit, exit 72, to the Zoo-Forestry Center.

From the airport: As you leave the airport, take the exit for I-205 south toward Portland. After a few miles, take the I-84 West exit, which also says Portland. Continue on toward downtown Portland, then exit on I-405 toward Beaverton. Head west on US 26, and after the tunnel, take the Zoo-Forestry Center exit, exit 72. It's about a 25-minute drive.

Public transportation: From the MAX light-rail: Get on the red/blue MAX line at Portland Pioneer Square. Exit at the Washington Park MAX station. This is the easiest way to arrive. The MAX line has geologic displays about its construction, and an art piece is on the Les AuCoin Memorial Plaza on the station side nearest the zoo. TriMet Bus 63 (Washington Park) stops at the World Forestry Center. Contact TriMet for information about fares and schedules (trimet.org).

Overview: Washington Park now covers 400 acres of the 5,100-acre Forest Park. The formal northeastern corner developed into a European style of park when prosperous Portlanders admired East Coast elegance. Frederick Law Olmsted's firm developed vistas and a master plan. The southwestern corner, a more-informal, child-accessible, and nature-oriented park, has a zoo, museums, the tranquil Vietnam Veteran's Memorial, and access to trails throughout Forest Park. The longest trail, Wildwood, begins here.

There are three separate elements in this walk. The first part covers the museum cluster around the central transportation plaza. The second is a peaceful reminder of the history and results of the Vietnam War. The third is a nature trail that gives a beginner a mile-long taste of trail experience. All three parts are handicapped-accessible, and can be done separately at different times.

The Walk

▶Start in front of the MAX light-rail station. Look south to see the Children's Museum. The Portland Zoo is to your left. The Discovery Museum building is directly in front of you.

▶Take the crosswalk across Knights Boulevard toward this building.

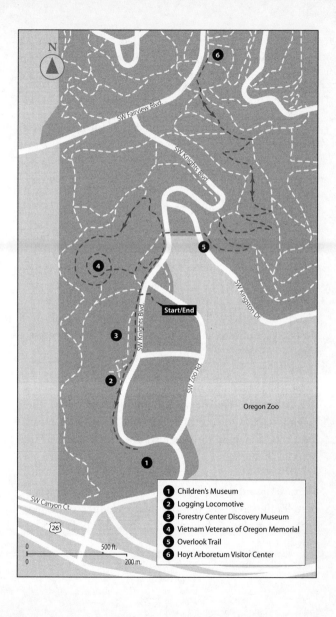

N

SW Fairview Blvd

SW Knights Blvd

6

4

5

SW Kingston Dr

SW Knights Blvd

Start/End

3

SW Zoo Rd

2

Oregon Zoo

1

SW Canyon Ct.

26

0	500 ft.
0	200 m.

1 Children's Museum
2 Logging Locomotive
3 Forestry Center Discovery Museum
4 Vietnam Veterans of Oregon Memorial
5 Overlook Trail
6 Hoyt Arboretum Visitor Center

▶Turn left on the sidewalk and go to the Children's Museum, whose motto is "The museum that doesn't act like a museum." Only adults accompanied by children are allowed beyond the museum lobby.

▶Outside the main entrance is the colorful *Kow for Kids* sculpture. Facing it from the sidewalk, go left to the east side of the building. Basalt boulders just the right size for children to climb on and use as hiding places are scattered across the lawn.

▶Return to the *Kow*. On your right is the Zany Maze—an outdoor maze tall enough for children to feel hidden, but short enough for parents to peer over. Admission to this is free.

▶Keep on the sidewalk passing the maze and walk north to the complex of buildings that make up the World Forestry Center.

▶Pass Merlo Hall and turn left by the Shay steam locomotive, designed to haul heavy loads on the steep and winding logging roads. On your right is a small sign commemorating David Douglas, the botanist. The tall Douglas fir tree bears his name.

▶Return toward the Shay steam locomotive. On your left are steps leading to a little platform where children can explore Peggy, the engine. A display sign in front tells of Peggy's logging history.

▶Go back to the sidewalk and turn left (north) to the World Forestry Center Discovery Museum. A handicapped-accessible ramp on your left winds around up to the building's entrance. Pass this, and continue past the flight of steps leading up to the museum's entrance.

WORLD FORESTRY CENTER DISCOVERY MUSEUM

The first Forestry Building was an enormous log cabin built from huge native trees displayed at the 1905 Lewis and Clark Centennial Exposition. It was so popular that the building was turned over to the State of Oregon. Fire destroyed it in 1964. This large wooden building was built in 1971 as the Western Forestry Center. Its name was later changed to World Forestry Center, with its emphasis on trees and forestry in all corners of the world.

Now there are several buildings, and this particular one is called the Discovery Museum. Inside are both permanent and interactive exhibits about the importance of forests and trees in our lives, as well as environmental sustainability. Appropriate for anyone from ages 3 to 103, visitors can take a whitewater raft ride without getting wet, ride up to the forest canopy, 50 feet above the forest floor, and take video journeys to Russia, China, South Africa, and Brazil, to learn about their forests and the challenges they face. The museum has a unique Forest Store with well-crafted and forest-related items, many made in Oregon.

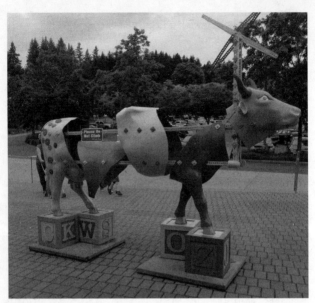

Kow for Kids greets all comers to the Children's Museum.

Dick Lukins

▶Walk past this building and follow the signs to the Vietnam Veterans of Oregon Memorial. This memorial is more than just a remembrance of our veterans; it also commemorates an important part of American culture and history.

▶Take the path on your left a few yards beyond some steps.

▶Turn onto the concrete walkway and go under a beautiful arched bridge. This takes you to a small fountain at the lovely Garden of Solace. Look up on the surrounding slopes to see the polished, black-granite memorial panels.

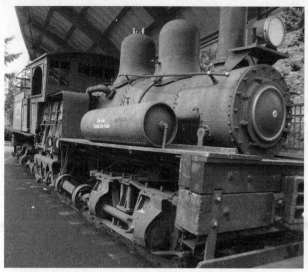

A locomotive lets you know you're in the right place.

Dick Lukins

The path on the left-hand side of the garden begins the gently spiraling walkway up to the walls. The path crosses the arched bridge, from which you can see another view of the fountain and garden. Trees and shrubs from the dogwood and rose families border the circular path.

▶Continue on the path until you arrive at the first wall commemorating the years 1959 to 1965. Take time to read the notes on each wall as you pass—they are excellent chronological reminders of recent American history, telling how we got into and out of this Cold War military conflict. This first wall represents the time during which the United States gradually intervened in the affairs of this former French colony, hoping to stop the spread of Communism. By 1965, the United States had 184,300 troops stationed in Vietnam.

▶Continue to the wall for 1966–67, the years in which the United States became increasingly involved. Note the increase in the number of names of the dead.

▶Go to the 1968–69 wall. During these years, North Vietnam began a major offensive, President Lyndon Johnson decided against reelection, and successor President Richard Nixon began increasing the air war. Names of Oregon casualties almost cover this wall.

▶Go to the wall for 1970–71. Antiwar protests were evidence of a growing desire to withdraw from Vietnam. The ground war was winding down.

▶Continue to the 1972–76 wall. North Vietnam occupied South Vietnam in 1975. The war was over. Only eleven names were added to the toll of Oregon dead during these years, but more than 1.5 million Vietnamese and Americans died in the ten years preceding.

▶Proceed to the final wall, listing all those Oregonians who were still missing in action in 1987. Stars mark the names of those whose remains have since been recovered.

▶Beyond this wall is the start of the short Dogwood Trail, which is not handicapped-accessible. Pick up the paved trail by returning to the memorial entrance and taking the left concrete walkway to a pedestrian crosswalk on Knights Boulevard. Cross this on the crosswalk to the parking lot. Otherwise, you can continue past the wall to the Dogwood Trail. A large interpretive sign will give you an overview of the many trails which crisscross the park.

▸Continue past this to the intersection with the Wildwood Trail. The 30-mile Wildwood Trail begins near here and winds through much of Forest Park, one of the larger parks in the United States. (This park is the setting for *Wildwood: The Wildwood Chronicles,* a 2011–13 fantasy series for children by Colin Meloy, illustrated by his wife Carson Ellis.)

▸Turn right on the Wildwood Trail and take it back down the hill to the trailhead at the pedestrian crosswalk on Knights Boulevard. Cross to the parking lot. The paved trail goes to your right along the south end of the parking lot.

▸Cross Kingston Boulevard at a second crosswalk to the signed and paved Overlook Trail. An interpretive sign here welcomes you to the Hoyt Arboretum. As you proceed up the hill to the right, notice the identification signs on posts and/or tree trunks.

▸Turn left (west) at the intersection of Overlook and Walnut Trails, staying on the paved path.

▸At the road, don't cross, but turn right (east) again and climb the gently sloped, paved switchbacks up the hill, enjoying the vistas over the southwest Portland hills gradually coming into view.

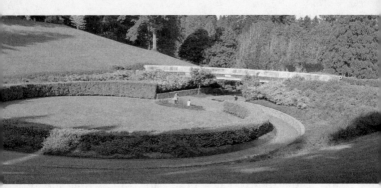

The Vietnam Memorial offers a space for quiet reflection. *Dick Lukins*

▸Pass some graveled steps as the paved path approaches the crest of the hill.

▸Proceed straight ahead on the Overlook Trail to the intersection of the Cherry Trail at the crest of the hill. You are passing between two water-storage tanks, barely visible through the vegetation.

▸Turn left where the paved Overlook Trail meets up with the Wildwood Trail, and take the gentle downhill grade. Cross the parking entrance to the Hoyt Arboretum Visitor Center and Nature Store. Drinking water and restrooms are here. Inside the building you will find maps, a Nature Store, and a knowledgeable staff of volunteers.

▸To return via the accessible paved path, retrace your route to the small parking lot at the corner of SW Kingston and SW Knights Boulevard. To explore other routes, obtain an Arboretum trail map at the Visitor Center.

Walk 10: Hoyt Arboretum Evergreen Trail

General location: Hoyt Arboretum is on the west side of Portland. In 2012 the American Conifer Society named it a Conifer Reference Garden, one of only two in the western United States.

Special attractions: A sylvan retreat containing 237 species of conifers

Difficulty: Moderately easy dirt trail with one uphill section

Distance: 2 miles

Estimated time: 1.5 hours

Services: Water, picnic shelter, picnic tables, visitor center with exhibits, a horticultural library, and a small shop with tree-related gifts and books. A few snacks are also available. The wheelchair-accessible restrooms remain open until the park closes at 10 p.m.

Restrictions: The center is staffed by volunteers and is generally open each day. Visitors are prohibited from picking any plants. No fires or alcoholic beverages are allowed in the park. Mountain bikes and motorized vehicles are prohibited on the trails.

For more information: Contact the Hoyt Arboretum (hoyt arboretum.org).

Getting started: From downtown Portland, take US 26 westbound to the Zoo-Forestry Center exit. Follow the signs to the Hoyt Arboretum Visitor Center at 4000 SW Fairview Boulevard. You can also take Burnside Street west to the arboretum by following the entrance sign on the left, about a mile west of NW 23rd. Keep following the signs to the arboretum. The main parking lot is on the south side of the visitor center.

Public transportation: Bus 63 (Washington Park) from downtown Portland stops at the Hoyt Arboretum Visitor Center. Contact TriMet for information about schedules and fares (trimet.org).

Overview: Stroll through the largest assortment of conifers in the world and see various species of redwood, spruce, fir, cedar, and pine. The Hoyt Arboretum features more than 800 labeled species of trees and shrubs spread out over 175 acres. There are 8 miles of trails within the arboretum itself, and some of these connect with other trails in Forest Park. Guided weekend nature walks are offered from April through October.

This was once the original site of the Multnomah County poor farm. Now it is a scientific garden and tree museum, as well as a public park. When the arboretum was established in 1931, its founders saved as many of the natural trees as possible. As plants from every continent of the world except Antarctica were added, they were carefully interspersed among the natives.

The Evergreen Trail combines sections of four trails into one walk among the evergreens of the Northwest. Open pine and spruce forests contrast with the denser growth of the coastal redwoods. *Meet the Trees,* an illustrated trail map designed for children, is available in the visitor center, and provides a good idea of what you may see. Several trails combine on this walk: Spruce, Wildwood, Creek, and Redwood.

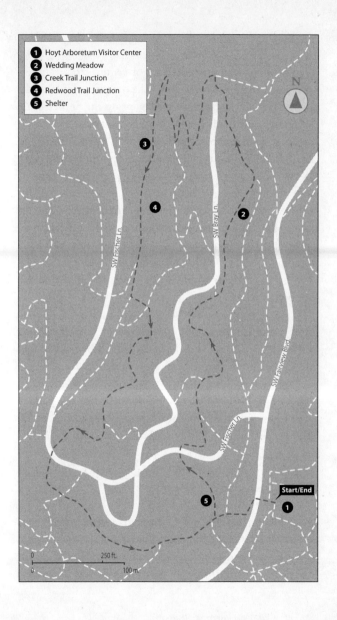

1 Hoyt Arboretum Visitor Center
2 Wedding Meadow
3 Creek Trail Junction
4 Redwood Trail Junction
5 Shelter

N

3
4
2

SW Fischer Ln
SW Bray Ln
SW Fairview Blvd
SW Fischer Ln

5
Start/End
1

0   250 ft.
0   100 m

The Walk

▶From the front door of the visitor center, cross Fairview Boulevard at the crosswalk and take the ramp down to the picnic shelter. The conifer tour begins on the Spruce Trail, to the right of the shelter's drinking fountain.

You'll pass some low-growing salal bushes. Birds and small mammals eat the purple berries, and it was food for the local Native Americans.

▶The Spruce Trail goes to the left of these bushes. Pass by some Manchurian firs before coming to a Douglas fir. The cones of this tree hang down from the branches, instead of standing upright, and botanists do not consider it to be a true fir. Douglas fir is one of the most preferred trees for lumber.

▶Look at one of the cones. Can you see the bracts sticking out from the scales? They have been described as the tails of mice sheltering from an Oregon rain.

▶Cross SW Fischer Lane and continue down the path to your right, past the Himalayan spruce. Stay to the left on the Spruce Trail, as another trail comes in from the right.

▶Pass a grove of spruce with a memorial bench. The Spruce Trail sign is across from the bench.

▶Go straight and then left through a grove of Norway spruce. Pass a knobcone pine. Take the path to your right at a fork and come out on the south side of the "Wedding Meadow." This is a popular spot for weddings because all the flowering plants here have white blossoms. Pass the star magnolia.

▶A bench remembering "Sniffles" is by the ponderosa pine on your right. Continue left on the Spruce Trail, ignoring the Yellow Pine Trail. Chinese black pines are just past some steps to the right.

▶Pass three exotic-looking weeping sequoias. One creeps along the ground near three upright ones. These trees are often used in landscaping, since no two trees ever look alike.

The Spruce Trail meets the Wildwood Trail, a popular jogging trail.

▶Go straight on the Wildwood Trail as it turns left downhill to a viewing platform and a grove of redwoods. Look up to see the height of these giant sequoias and coast redwoods. You may hear birds singing and smell the trees' distinct fragrance.

▶Return to the Wildwood Trail and proceed down the switchbacks. Pass a memorial bench for two beloved dogs.

▶Turn right at the intersection to the Redwood Trail and continue on this until you reach a footbridge. Do not cross the bridge but continue straight on the Creek Trail.

▶Pass a grove of yellow cedar. Continue on the trail, crossing the creek twice.

▶Stay to the left at the fork in the trail. A tree with a totally exposed root system is on the hillside to your left.

▶Proceed to a footbridge.

▶Turn left and climb some steps up to the Redwood Trail. Turn right.

▶Pass several Cedars of Lebanon before entering a grove of Atlas cedar.

▶Go right at the trail fork, continuing on the Redwood Trail.

▶Cross SW Fischer Lane, watching carefully for traffic.

▶Proceed uphill through a grove of Japanese larches.

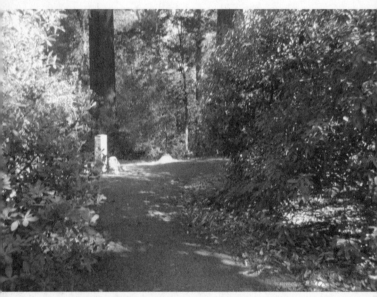

Shady trails wind through the arboretum.

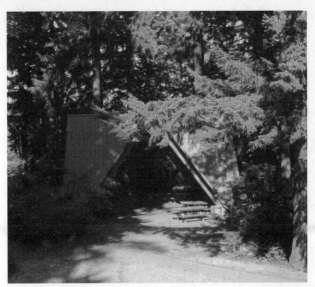
A picnic shelter is near the entrance of the Evergreen Walk.

▶Cross a trail intersection and pass the memorial bench for John M. Bond. The path continues uphill to your right through a variety of hemlocks and firs. You will pass a tall noble fir.

▶Go left at the Fir Trail junction. The picnic shelter is just ahead.

▶Turn right at the shelter and return across Fairview Boulevard to the visitor center.

Walk 11: Hoyt Arboretum Bristlecone Trail

General location: Hoyt Arboretum is 2 miles west of Portland

Special attractions: This is a gently sloping trail, wheelchair-accessible, that gives a close-up view of the world's largest collection of conifers.

Difficulty: Easy and paved

Distance: 0.5 mile

Estimated time: 30 minutes

Services: The visitor center has exhibits, a horticultural library, and a small shop with tree-related gifts and books. A few snacks are also available. Drinking fountains and wheelchair-accessible restrooms are outside, along with picnic tables and a shelter.

Restrictions: The wheelchair-accessible restrooms are open until the park closes at 10 p.m. Visitors are prohibited from picking plants. No fires or alcoholic beverages are allowed in the park. Mountain bikes and motorized vehicles are prohibited on the trails.

For more information: Contact the Hoyt Arboretum, 4000 SW Fairview Boulevard, Portland, OR 97221; (503) 865-8733; hoytarboretum.org.

Getting started: From downtown Portland, take US 26 westbound to the Zoo-Forestry Center exit. Follow the signs to the Hoyt Arboretum Visitor Center at 4000 SW Fairview Boulevard. You can also take Burnside Street west to the arboretum by following the entrance sign on the left, about a mile west of NW 23rd. Keep following the signs to the arboretum. The main parking lot is on the south side of the visitor center, but there is also parking at the Bristlecone trailhead.

To reach the Bristlecone trailhead from the arboretum parking lot, turn right onto SW Fairview Boulevard. Take the first left onto SW Fischer Lane. Drive or walk down this lane for 0.2 miles. The Bristlecone Trail parking area is on your left.

Public transportation: Bus 63 (Washington Park) from downtown Portland stops at the Hoyt Arboretum Visitor Center. Contact TriMet for information about fares and schedules (trimet.org).

Overview: This paved path takes you through a variety of conifers, with benches and viewpoints along the way to help you enjoy the route.

The Walk

►A basalt rock wall and several bristlecone specimens mark the trailhead on the north side of the parking lot. Start up the trail to your right, toward a large monkey puzzle tree on your left. The curls at the end of the long branches resemble monkey tails. A weathered bench and moss-covered boulders are on your left at the top of the hill. The trail loops around a large Douglas fir. Pacific dogwood trees are on your right.

►Where two trails come together, take the one on your right, turning past a grand fir. Enter a canopy of vine

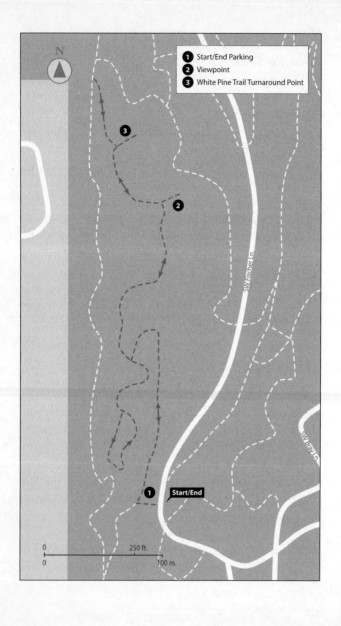

1 Start/End Parking
2 Viewpoint
3 White Pine Trail Turnaround Point

Start/End

SW Fischer Ln

SW Bray Ln

0   250 ft.
0   100 m.

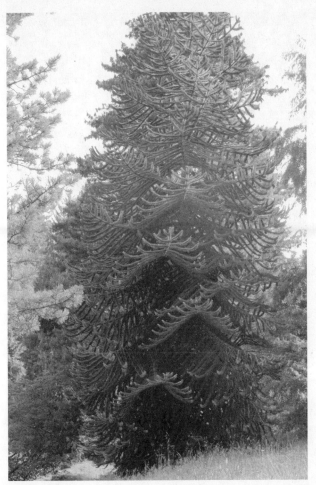

Do you think these branches look like monkey tails?

Dick Lukins

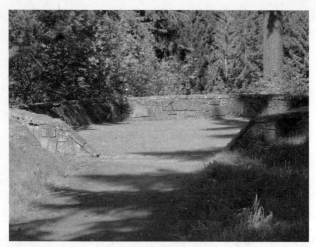

The trail is paved for handicapped access. *Dick Lukins*

maples. A bench in memory of Martha Biggs sits by a little drainage rivulet with more mossy boulders.

▶Continue on the path past another bench in memory of Ruth Hyde, and past a grove of paper birch. From here, you can look across a little valley to a forested hill.

▶Continue on the trail. On your right a large stone circle provides a pleasant place for sitting or picnicking.

▶Return to the trail, continuing right. You will pass a maidenhair ginkgo on your right. Other types of ginkgoes are also found in this area.

▶Continue until the paving ends at the junction with the gravel White Pine Trail. This pleasant clearing with picnic tables is your turnaround spot. When you are ready to leave, go back the way you came, down the paved hill.

▸When you come to the junction of two trails at the grand fir and the noble fir, keep to your right on the paved trail. Take the path past white fir and cypress. Pass the Vizzini memorial bench by the red-barked madrone tree.

▸At a second fork in the paved path, go right again. A weathered bench at the end of the paved path overlooks Fischer Lane.

▸Circle back to the right through a beech grove and return down the trail to the starting point in the parking lot.

SOUTHWEST

Walk 12: South Portland—Lair Hill Neighborhood

📷 ✕ 🏢

General location: South of the Ross Island Bridge and on both sides of I-5

Special attractions: Nicely restored, century-old homes in one of Portland's original neighborhoods, and three different neighborhood parks

Difficulty: Moderate; a hilly area with old sidewalks and narrow streets

Distance: 3 miles

Estimated time: 1.5 hours

Services: Restrooms and water are available at the Duniway and Lair Hill Parks.

Restrictions: Dogs must be leashed.

For more information: Contact the Portland Oregon Visitors Association, 701 SW 6th Avenue, Portland, OR 97204; (503) 275-8355; travelportland.com; or South Waterfront Community Relations, 0841 SW Gaines Street, Suite #115, Portland, OR 97239; (503) 972-3289; southwaterfront.com.

Getting started: From downtown Portland go to SW Clay Street and Naito Parkway. Head west on Clay, and turn left onto SW 5th Avenue. Cross US 26 and turn left onto

SW Sheridan Street. Turn left onto SW 4th Avenue, which becomes SW Barbur Boulevard. The Travelodge is at 2401 Barbur Boulevard, on the corner of Barbur Boulevard and Caruthers Street.

Public transportation: Buses 44 and 12 travel north and south on 4th Street.

Overview: Lair Hill is named not for a hill but for a man, William Lair Hill. This is the west section of the historic South Portland neighborhood. Families coming along the Oregon Trail and single men seeking business opportunities in Portland settled here before the Civil War. Many young men traveled by sea around South America.

Another wave of immigration came in near the turn of the century. These immigrants were mostly from Europe, and the area became known as "Little Italy" and "Little Russia" because of their home countries. They took pride in their modest homes, imitating the Victorian architecture of the hilltop mansions. Two family homes were designed to look like one large home with a single flight of stairs and large front porch. Mass production of building components made it possible to individualize homes with decorative woodwork. Most of the houses in this—and the Corbett—neighborhood were built between 1880 and 1920.

As the initial settlers and their families moved away, the remaining buildings in South Portland were beginning to show their age and need of repair. In the1960s an urban renewal project demolished the northern part of the neighborhood near the city's core. Freeways for automobiles, with little respect for pedestrians or community, sliced the remains of South Portland into three separate pieces: Lair Hill, Corbett, and South Waterfront.

Lair Hill residents persuaded the city to establish a Historic Conservation District for this south part of Portland in1975, dedicating the area to "developing a sense of community" in an effort to maintain the original quality of this working-class neighborhood. Corbett-area residents followed suit. New owners now vie to restore these houses to their original glory. As you meander through the area, every street boasts delightful examples of paint, exterior trims, and design.

As Portland grew, so did its waterfront. By World War I, the farmland in what is now known as the South Waterfront had become an industrial and shipbuilding area. Shipbuilding continued in World War II, after which it was used for ship dismantling and barge building. The area was designated as a polluted "brownfield," and named an urban renewal project.

Today's urban planning encourages high-density living with open spaces, sustainability, and transportation by foot, bike, and streetcar. Oregon Health and Science University (OHSU) planned an outpatient facility on the waterfront. The city built an aerial tram to connect with the main hospitals and other facilities on Marquam Hill. Today you will find the Willamette River is a major asset, encouraging a sense of openness and neighborly interchange among the high-rises. Such pedestrian-friendly features as small shops and businesses, a well-planned park, a community garden, and an unleashed dog park also bring residents together in day-to-day connections. The new Hooley Pedestrian Bridge at Gibbs Street connects these two parts of Portland, and plans have been drawn up for a future connection across Naito Parkway. Then, once again, you will be able to do a complete walk through all South Portland neighborhoods.

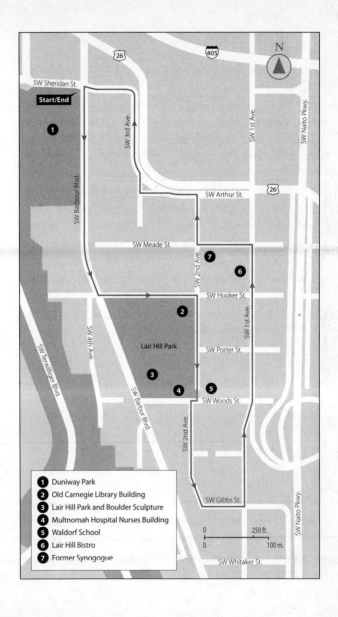

SW Sheridan St.

Start/End

I-405

US 26

N

1 Duniway Park

SW Barbur Blvd

SW 3rd Ave.

SW 1st Ave.

SW Naito Pkwy.

SW Arthur St.

US 26

SW Meade St.

7 Former Synagogue

6 Lair Hill Bistro

SW 2nd Ave.

SW Hooker St.

2 Old Carnegie Library Building

SW 4th Ave.

Lair Hill Park

SW 1st Ave.

SW Porter St.

SW Terwilliger Blvd.

3 Lair Hill Park and Boulder Sculpture

4 Multnomah Hospital Nurses Building

5 Waldorf School

SW Woods St.

SW Barbur Blvd.

SW 2nd Ave.

SW Gibbs St.

1	Duniway Park
2	Old Carnegie Library Building
3	Lair Hill Park and Boulder Sculpture
4	Multnomah Hospital Nurses Building
5	Waldorf School
6	Lair Hill Bistro
7	Former Synagogue

0   250 ft.
0   100 m.

SW Whitaker St.

SW Naito Pkwy.

The Walk

▸Begin at the Travelodge Hotel, 2401 SW 4th Avenue and Caruthers Street.

▸Go south through the parking lot on the corner of Sheridan and 4th. You may park here or at Duniway Park on the other side of Sheridan.

▸Turn right to the crosswalk across Sheridan Street, and cross to Duniway Park, named for Abigail Scott Duniway, who came from Illinois on the Oregon Trail in 1851. She became a famous women's rights advocate, and when Oregon women won the right to vote in 1912, the governor asked her to write and sign the equal suffrage proclamation.

▸Continue south to Hooker Street, passing a former YMCA building and parking lot.

▸Turn left and cross Barbur at the signal. Walk east on Hooker. On your right is Lair Hill Park, named for William Lair Hill, who bought the property in 1868 but never lived there. Hill was born in Tennessee and moved to Oregon in 1853. He was an attorney, historian, and newspaper editor, remembered for his work codifying Oregon law and establishing parks in Portland.

▸On the corner of 2nd Avenue, note the Italian Renaissance Revival building on the corner. Built in 1921, this was originally the Carnegie Branch Library. In front of the building is a huge copper beech tree, probably brought as a seed from Germany.

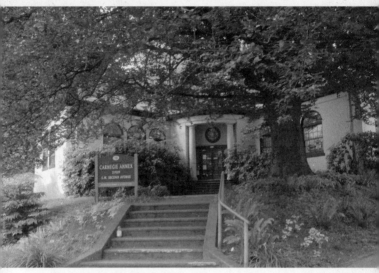

This copper beech is thought to have come from Germany.

▸Walk south on 2nd Avenue. The 3-acre Lair Hill Park is located on the west side of 2nd. Note the gate where you can enter the park and view the beautiful heritage trees. At the west end of the park, a sculpture of metal boulders by local artist Bruce West represents the rock grotto which once stood in the park, providing a shady place where older men would gather on hot summer days to play chess. It was installed in 1978.

▸Continue south into the closed-off portion of the street that now serves as the courtyard of the Cedarwood Waldorf School, on your left. This 1904 brick building, designed by A. E. Doyle and known as the Neighborhood House, was one of the centers of the community. It served Eastern

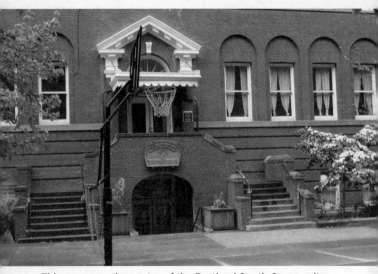

This was once the center of the Portland South Community.

European Jewish immigrants, teaching them to read, write, and speak English, and to learn other skills necessary for citizenship. It is listed on the National Register of Historic Places. Across the courtyard in the southern corner of the park is another brick building. This Georgian Revival house was built in 1918 as a dormitory for Multnomah County Hospital nurses. It later served as the Children's Museum before that institution moved to its present location near the Zoo.

▶Exit the courtyard, cross Woods Street, and continue on the west side of 2nd Avenue. Before crossing Grover Street, you will see on your left some classic box-style row houses, built in 1906 (numbers 3122, 3124, 3132, and 3138). On your right—number 3025, just before the road curves to your left—is a Victorian with an impressive outdoor stairway to the second floor.

▸Stay left as the road passes an imposing tile-roofed building. Follow it around to 1st Avenue. Since the trolley ran along this street, it was a more commercial road.

▸Turn left and proceed north on 1st Avenue, passing a brick building that once was a car garage and brass factory. It is now the office of Walsh Construction Company. Note the

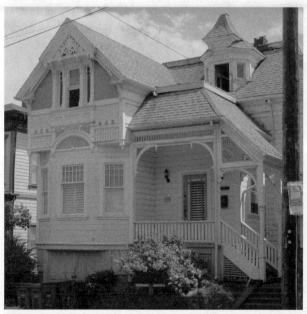

Haehlen House is a lovely example of Italianate Victorian architecture.

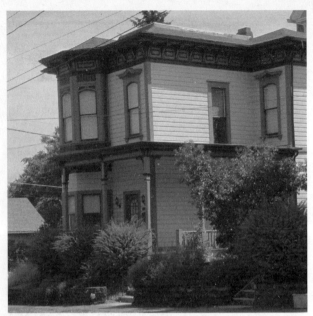

Peter Taylor also built the Peter Taylor House next door.

two hammers on either side of the entrance. The sign on the building explains the symbolism. Continue toward Woods. This high Victorian at 3101 SW 1st Avenue was built around 1889 and served as an immigrant apartment house. It was one of the first houses in the neighborhood to be renovated.

▶Continue north, crossing Woods and Porter. Cross Hooker and continue to the Lair Hill Bistro. Stop and look east across 1st Avenue. Two historic houses are here. The pink-and-white Italianate Victorian at number 2818 was the home of John and Gotlieb Haehlen, who came to Portland from Lenk, Switzerland. It was originally built by Peter Taylor and sold to the Haehlens. Note the intricate details in the trim and the little door in the tower. This house is often considered one the best examples of this style in Portland.

Next to it at number 2806 is the Peter Taylor House, built in 1882, and one of the two oldest structures in the area. Taylor, a blacksmith, came by the Oregon Trail and arrived in Portland in 1853. He worked at the Oregon Iron Works, and then founded the Willamette Iron Works, which produced many of the cast-iron building fronts in downtown Portland.

The Lair Hill Bistro is one of the dozens of businesses that once lined this street. It is still family-owned and functions as a restaurant and bar. Note the living quarters above the Bistro, a common practice at the time.

▶Cross Meade, continuing north on 1st Street. The nicely painted Victorian at 2737 SW 1st Avenue was built in the 1880s, and was later owned by the family of Earl Riley, mayor of Portland during World War II. Originally located five blocks to the south, near the fire station where Riley's father worked, it was moved to the present site in 1979. Note the solar-heating panel on the south-facing roof.

Across the street from the Riley House is the small house built by Philip Augustus Marquam, who was called "the greatest landowner in Multnomah County." Born in Baltimore, he graduated from law school and arrived in Portland in 1851. He acquired a great deal of land, including the property now known as Marquam Hill (or "Pill Hill," because of the hospitals situated on top). Many Portland buildings were named after him.

▸Return to Meade Street, cross, and turn to your right (west). The building at 116 SW Meade, now a private residence, was built in 1913 as the original South Portland Branch Library. It was so heavily used that a new Carnegie library had to be opened in 1923. The residents carried the books, uphill, to the new library in Lair Hill Park.

▸Pass the beautiful, restored, yellow Queen Anne house with the garage underneath. Across Meade is the Anna B. Crocker House. She was a portrait artist. Note that the house is very close to the sidewalk, with no front yard.

▸Go to the pale green building on the corner. Note the stained-glass windows, the Gothic vestigial buttresses on the side, and the crenellations on the top. Built as a Baptist church in 1881, it was purchased by three Eastern European Jews in 1912 and became the Meade Street Shul. It then became the (Orthodox) Kesser Israel Synagogue. Now it is the home of the evangelical New Church of All Nations.

▸At 2nd avenue, turn right and cross Meade. The house on this corner, numbers 2737 and 2740, was built by John Corkish, an Irish immigrant from the Isle of Man. Note the two covered bins on the south side of the house, designed for putting coal into the basement. This beautifully restored Queen Anne–style building, known as the Corkish Apartments, is listed on the National Register because of its historic and architectural significance.

▸The two houses on the west side of the street, numbers 2723 and 2731, were built in 1880 and 1908, and were later occupied by the Zidell Family. Sam Zidell emigrated from Kiev, Russia (now Ukraine), and arrived in Portland in 1915. In the early years, the Zidell family was in the scrap-metal business, and by 1946 they were the nation's largest ship dismantlers. They are still operating today on the South Waterfront as builders of double-hulled steel barges.

▶Continue down 2nd Street to Arthur.

▶Turn left on Arthur. Walk up the hill and turn right on 3rd to Sheridan. Turn left to Barbur Boulevard, crossing with the traffic signal, and turn right to return to your starting point at the Travelodge, or Duniway Park.

Walk 13: South Portland— Corbett Neighborhood

General location: South of the Ross Island Bridge and on both sides of I-5

Special attractions: Nicely restored, century-old homes in one of Portland's original neighborhoods, nearby high-rises in Oregon's first green neighborhood, and a new pedestrian bridge over I-5, tying the two together

Difficulty: Moderately difficult; a hilly area with old sidewalks and narrow streets

Distance: 3 miles

Estimated time: 1.5 hours

Services: Restrooms are in the OHSU building. If closed, there is a porta-potty opposite on the east side of Bond Street.

Restrictions: OHSU's Health and Healing Center is open Monday through Friday, 8 a.m. to 6 p.m.

For more information: Contact the River's Edge Hotel and Spa, 455 SW Hamilton Court, Portland, OR 97239; (503) 802-5800; or South Waterfront Community Relations, 0841 SW Gaines Street, Suite #115, Portland, OR 97239; (503) 972-3289; southwaterfront.com.

Getting started: Reach the River's Edge Hotel and Spa, 0455 SW Hamilton Court, from Macadam Avenue. To reach Macadam Avenue from the north, take I-5 south. Take exit 299A toward Lake Oswego. Take slight right on SW Macadam Avenue OR 43. Turn left at the first signal onto Hamilton Court.

From the south, take I-5 North. Take the Corbett Road exit, exit 298, and turn right onto SW Corbett Avenue. Turn left onto SW Macadam Avenue. Turn right into SW Hamilton Court.

Public transportation: Buses 35 Macadam/Greeley, and 36 South Shore also stop in the area. Check with TriMet (trimet.org) for current information. The N-S line Portland streetcar stops at Lowell Street. From there walk south a half-mile along the Moody trolley tracks to Hamilton Street, and turn left to the River's Edge Hotel and Spa

Overview: The Corbett and Lair Hill walks go through a large collection of historic working-class homes dating from the late 1800s to the early part of the twentieth century. This area, once considered a slum, was saved from urban renewal by residents who were appalled at what had happened to the northern part of the community. But the major highways slicing through it left most roads as dead ends, making it difficult for developers to navigate. Left to itself, it was later rediscovered by a new generation who appreciated the large trees and charming structures of the original small houses. Today these homes are being carefully painted and restored, and every street has interesting examples of architecture.

The South Waterfront area is a total contrast. Originally farmland for the houses on the hill, it underwent years of industrial pollution. Once plans were made to clean up the Willamette and its neighborhoods, this was planned to be a green, sustainable, high-density, and walkable area, relying on public transportation systems rather than cars. The OHSU building anchors the neighborhood, and the waterfront provides a focal point for nearly every building. This is still a work in progress, and the neighborhood

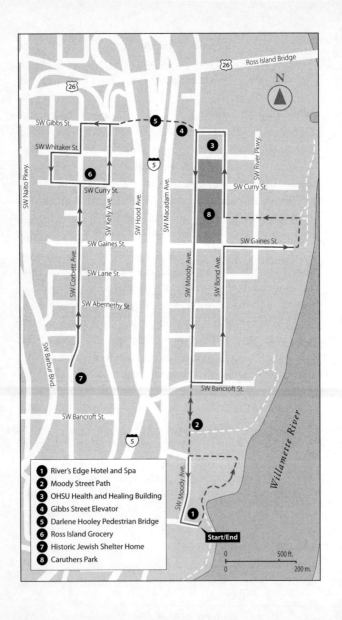

SW Naito Pkwy.

SW Gibbs St.

SW Whitaker St.

SW Curry St.

SW Kelly Ave.

SW Hood Ave.

SW Macadam Ave.

SW River Pkwy.

SW Curry St.

SW Gaines St.

SW Corbett Ave.

SW Gaines St.

SW Lane St.

SW Abernethy St.

SW Moody Ave.

SW Bond Ave.

SW Barbur Blvd.

SW Bancroft St.

SW Bancroft St.

SW Moody Ave.

Willamette River

Ross Island Bridge

N

1 River's Edge Hotel and Spa
2 Moody Street Path
3 OHSU Health and Healing Building
4 Gibbs Street Elevator
5 Darlene Hooley Pedestrian Bridge
6 Ross Island Grocery
7 Historic Jewish Shelter Home
8 Caruthers Park

Start/End

0   500 ft.

0   200 m.

community has a positive feeling about the future. The 2012 Hooley Pedestrian Bridge now ties the Corbett and South Waterfront neighborhoods together.

The Walk

▶Leave the River's Edge Hotel and Spa and turn left through the posts to the path between the hotel and the Aquariva restaurant. Turn left as the path joins the greenway along the river.

▶Keep north as it passes the redbrick River Forum building. It turns left around the end of the building, going west up a slight hill to the parking lot.

▶The path turns right just before the trolley tracks. Keep them on your left. The tracks and the path end at Bancroft Street.

▶Turn right on Bancroft. Pass a charter school and a storage building. You'll see a stop sign just before the parking lot for the Old Spaghetti Factory. Cross River Parkway and turn left.

▶Go one long block to Gaines Street and turn right toward the river.

▶Turn left on the brick path behind Atwater Place (waterfront condos). The greenway to your right along the river is presently undergoing renovation, but this path gives an equally good view of the river and of Ross Island.

▸Take the first left into a wide pedestrian walkway. This is Pennoyer, once a through street. Atwater Place is now on your left. Cross River Parkway, and go one more block to Bond Avenue. You may find a vehicle or two parking on this section of Pennoyer.

▸Turn right on Bond. The building on your right is the Mirabella, one of the first vertical retirement communities in the nation. Pass the pools and small courtyard at the entrance, and notice the large aluminum and art glass harp-like flower. A tiny frog climbs up the back. Across Bond Avenue is Elizabeth Caruthers Park, named for the pioneer woman who came on the Oregon Trail in 1847. She lived and farmed with her son, Finice, on their donation land claims that are now the South Waterfront and Corbett neighborhoods. After her death, many tried to take her property, saying a single woman could not own a donation land claim. The US Supreme Court upheld this right.

▸Cross Curry and then cross Bond. Turn right, toward the OHSU's Center for Health and Healing Building. The grassy lawn on your left is the roof of the underground parking garage.

▸Cross Whitaker, pass the OHSU building, and turn the corner. The entrance to the overhead tram is on your right.

▸Continue straight to the Gibbs Street traffic signal and cross Moody to the small plaza. The tall, thin building in front of you is an elevator up to the Darlene Hooley Pedestrian Bridge, named for the congresswoman who helped arrange for federal funding. This steel box girder bridge crosses busy Macadam Avenue and I-5, restoring the ties between the Corbett area and the South Waterfront. The pull-through elevator is large enough for bikes with trailers, and the energetic can take a 132-step stairway with bike trough up to the bridge.

▸Choose your route up to the bridge and its viewing platform, designed to resemble the prow of a ship. If you choose the elevator, notice the varied photographic water patterns on the glass as you ascend. Walk straight across the 700-foot concrete bridge to the western side. You will exit at Kelly Avenue, entering the Corbett neighborhood at Gibbs and Kelly. The Corbett neighborhood was named for Henry W. Corbett, one of many young men who sailed around "The Horn" from Massachusetts in 1851. He became a businessman and influential politician, and served as a US senator from 1867 to 1873.

▸Cross Kelly and go straight west on Gibbs for one block. This is Corbett Avenue. In some places there are no street signs, but these old neighborhoods have street names stamped into the concrete sidewalks at the corners. This is no longer done, but the city tries to maintain this signage.

▸Turn right on Corbett Avenue and walk north. The fourth building on your right down the hill, #3204, is one of the oldest in the area, having been built in 1876. It was originally a boardinghouse for many of the Hebrew School teachers.

▸Return up the hill on Corbett, cross Gibbs, and walk south to Whitaker.

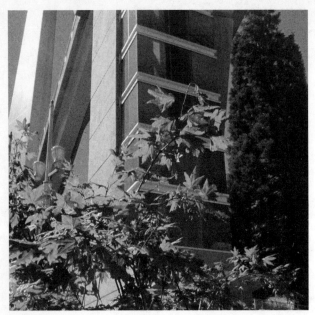
The elevator has room for bikes pulling trailers.

▶Turn right on Whitaker and then left on Water Avenue. Note the four row houses on the east side of Water's 3400 block, identical in structure but totally different in appearance. The southernmost house has a Povey stained-glass transom, with the former house number above the door, an expensive decoration. Brothers John and David Povey learned about the design and manufacture of stained-glass windows from their father, an immigrant from England. Their business, located in downtown Portland, installed distinctive stained-glass windows in churches and homes in Portland and other cities in Oregon, beginning in 1889.

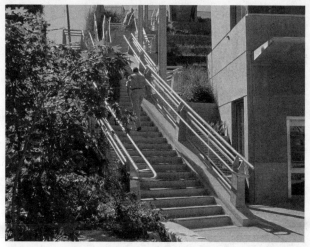

The stairs by the elevator building have troughs for bicycles.

▶Turn left on Curry and walk one block to Corbett Avenue. The Ross Island Grocery is an old business but recently moved to this new site. Besides groceries, it now functions as a deli and coffee shop.

SIDE TRIP

From here you may take an optional trip of seven blocks south on Corbett. At 4133 Corbett, the house with a rounded front porch is the Jewish Shelter Home. Elmer Cromwell, an Oregon legislator, built this home in 1902. It was purchased in 1919 by seventy-eight-year-old Jeanette Meier as a home for Jewish children whose families were unable to care for them. Jeanette Meier's son, Julius Meier, founded the Meier

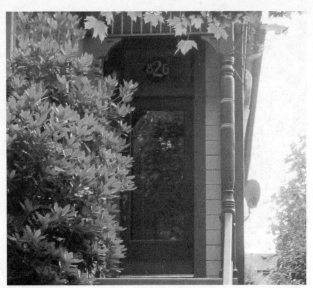

The old street number is centered in this Povey stained-glass window.

& Frank Department Store (now Macy's) in downtown Portland. Meier & Frank board meetings were often held at this site. Note the beautiful landscaping.

Retrace your steps on 4133 Corbett to Lane Street. On the way back, note the small pink house with the large bird weathervane at 4126. Cross and stop at the corner. Look west. The beautiful old oak you see is the Corbett Oak. Neighbors rallied to keep developers from razing this old oak by buying the tree and the lot and giving it to the city as Heritage Tree Park at Corbett and Lane.

End your side trip by continuing on Corbett to the Ross Island Grocery.

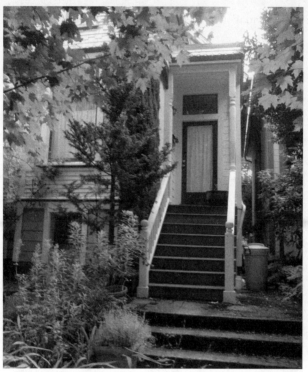

Even row houses have their own personalities. *Dick Lukins*

▶Turn right on Curry. Walk one block east to Kelly Avenue. Cross to the northeast intersection. The building at the corner, #3434, is the Milton Smith residence, a very handsome Colonial Revival building. This residence, built in 1891–92, is thought to be the first in the area to be wired for electricity. It is listed on the National Register of Historic Places, both because of its historic integrity and its associations with the architectural firm of Whidden & Lewis, designers of the historic Portland

Hotel and Portland City Hall, and employer of A. E. Doyle.

▶Continue north to the Henry Weinhard House at the 3400 corner of Whitaker. Weinhard was born in Germany, apprenticed in the brewing trade in Stuttgart, and immigrated to the United States. He came to Portland in 1862. He was obviously a smart marketer; when the elegant Skidmore Fountain was unveiled in 1887, he offered to pump in free beer. (The offer was declined.) By 1990 his Portland brewery was considered the largest in the Northwest. It relocated to Hood River as the Blitz-Weinhard Brewery, and some brewery remnants are now part of the Brewery Blocks condominium complex on West Burnside Street in Portland. Henry Weinhard also lived for a while on SW 2nd Avenue in the Lair Hill neighborhood.

▶Cross Whitaker and continue on Kelly until you reach Gibbs. Turn right and take the Pedestrian Bridge east across the eleven lanes of traffic beneath the bridge. Stop to enjoy the gorgeous view of the river and Mount Hood before returning to Moody Street. Use the traffic signal to cross Moody.

▶Turn right and continue south, crossing Whitaker, passing Caruthers Park, and cross Gaines. Pass the Riva on the Park Apartments on your left. Cross Abernathy and look right to see the old Moody docks, now home to some of Portland's ubiquitous food carts.

▶Pass the Matisse Apartments, cross Lowell, and pass the Gray's Landing building. When you reach Bancroft, cross to the path by the trolley tracks. Notice the sign saying BANCROFT STATION. This was once a stop on a narrow-gauge steam railroad that ran from Portland to Oswego, and which later became the Willamette Shore trolley. At present this portion is now unused, although there are efforts to reinstate it to ease car traffic on Macadam.

▶Continue south on the path. Go straight on Moody past the parking lots, and pass the trees and plantings along the west walls of the River's Edge Hotel and Spa lawn area. The tracks are on your right.

▶Turn left at Hamilton Court to your starting point at the entrance to the River's Edge Hotel and Spa.

Walk 14: Willamette Greenway

📷 ✕ 👫 🍃 ♿

General location: The southwest section of Portland

Special attractions: View the varied traffic on the Willamette River, Willamette Park, Butterfly Park, marinas, and John's Landing

Difficulty: Easy, on a paved walking/bike path

Distance: 3 miles

Estimated time: 2 hours

Services: Restrooms and water in Willamette Park

Restrictions: Note the signs where private property owners have granted access.

For more information: portlandoregon.gov/transportation.

Getting started: Reach the River's Edge Hotel and Spa, 0455 SW Hamilton Court, from Macadam Avenue. To reach Macadam Avenue from the north, take I-5 South. Take exit 299A toward Lake Oswego. Take slight right on SW Macadam OR 43. Turn left at the first signal onto Hamilton Court.

From the south, take I-5 North. Take the Corbett Road exit, exit 298, and turn right onto SW Corbett Avenue. Turn left onto SW Macadam Avenue. Turn right onto SW Hamilton Court. Valet parking is free during the day.

Public transportation: Buses 35 Macadam/Greeley, and 36 South Shore also stop in the area. Check with TriMet (trimet.org) for current information. The N-S Portland streetcar stops at Lowell Street. From there walk south a half-mile along the Moody trolley tracks to Hamilton Street and turn left to the River's Edge Hotel and Spa.

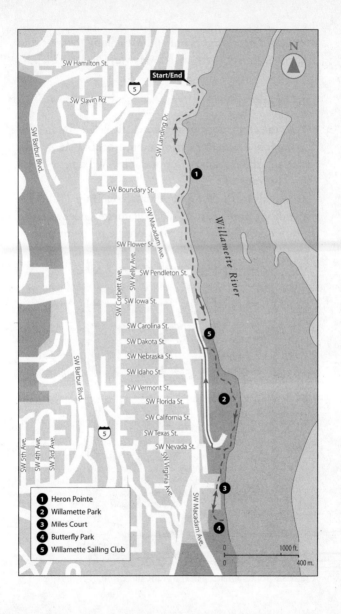

Overview: The walk goes out and back along the west side of the Willamette River, with lovely views of Ross Island.

The Walk

▸From the front door of the hotel, turn left toward the river and take walk/bike path around behind the hotel's restaurant, the Aquariva. Go south. The Willamette River will be on your left.

The path turns past a large office building. Although the path is public, part of the Willamette Greenway, the land on either side of the path is private property, part of

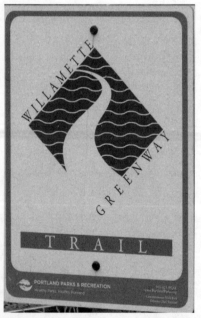

A marker points walkers in the right direction. *Dick Lukins*

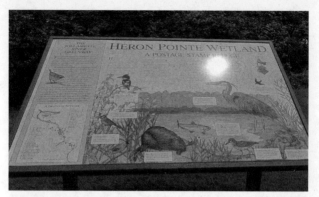

These signs tell about private owners' cooperation in wildlife preservation. *Dick Lukins*

the John's Landing development of condos, apartments, and townhouses. Stop at a bench by Heron Pointe and listen to the bird sounds. A Willamette Greenway display sign tells you about the plants and animals inhabiting this area. There is a small memorial plaque in the ground with a bronze statue of a beaver. Passersby often place sticks or flowers in his clasped hands.

▶Continue south on the bike path. You will see the marina for the John's Landing Boating Club on your left. Across the water is Ross Island, with a heron rookery and trees that provide nesting places for Canada geese. In front of it is tiny Toe Island, hard to see even when the water is low. A few small trees on top mark its location.

▶Turn left at the top of the path and go past the Willamette Sailing Club. The path then turns left back to the river. Stay on this path, as it goes through groves of trees and then comes out at the large parking lot for the public boat-launch area. On the far side of the parking lot are restrooms and a drinking fountain. This is Willamette Park, with soccer fields, tennis courts, and picnic tables.

The path continues on your left, passing two soccer fields and a very popular picnic shelter. You can see the tennis courts beyond.

▶Keep on the left and pass a third soccer field. Just beyond is a small children's play area with swings and teeter-totters.

▶Go through the posts and you will be on a small street, Miles Court. This was once part of a town named Fulton, which disappeared after the mills closed, and is one of the few remnants of the working-class homes that once filled the area. It is slowly becoming an area of newer homes, which take advantage of the river views.

▶Pass the homes and proceed through a grove of trees. Turn on the small path to your left, marked by some mossy boulders. This is the Butterfly Park Naturescape. Formerly a gravel parking lot and refuse area, volunteers began planting wildflower seeds from the Columbia Gorge here in 1991, and this lovely little area is the result.

▶Go to the bench by the river, where there is a memorial plaque for children installed by the Compassionate Friends. Then return on the bike path to Willamette Park.

▶Once through the posts and in the park, turn left and take Idaho Street. Pass the tennis courts. Keep on Idaho across Nebraska Street, where it becomes Beaver Avenue. Just beyond here the bike trail joins the road from the right.

▶Pass the Willamette Sailing Club. The Greenway path turns right just past the Sailing Club, and you can retrace your steps to the River's Edge Hotel and Spa. If you decide to return on a different route along a busier street, turn left on Carolina Street to Macadam Avenue just before the end of the Sailing Club property.

▶Turn right on Macadam Avenue. This street is busy, but offers an interesting mix of the old and the new in the way of shops, office buildings, restaurants, and apartments.

▶Cross Iowa Street and go three blocks to Boundary Road/ Landing Square. Turn toward the river, then left on Landing Drive. This road mainly serves condominium residents.

▶Keep on this road to your starting point at the River's Edge Hotel and Spa.

Walk 15: South Waterfront Parks

📷 ✕ 🚻 🏢 ♿

General location: Downtown Portland, west of I-5, South Waterfront District

Special attractions: Two twenty-first-century Portland parks

Difficulty: Easy, flat

Distance: 3 miles

Estimated time: 2 hours

Services: Restrooms and water in South Waterfront Park

Restrictions: The parks are open in the daytime. Dogs must be on a leash.

For more information: Portland Oregon Visitors Association, 701 Southwest 6th Avenue, Portland, OR 97204; (503) 275-8355; travelportland.com; or Portland Parks and Recreation, 1120 SW 5th Avenue #1302, Portland, OR 97204; (503) 823-7529; portlandonline.com/park; or the RiverPlace Hotel, 1510 Southwest Harbor Way, Portland, OR 97201; (503) 228-3233; riverplacehotel.com.

Getting started: From I-5 (southbound), take the exit to City Center / OMSI. Take the right lane and follow signs to Morrison Street/Bridge. Stay in the right lane on Morrison Bridge. Take the Naito Parkway exit and loop onto Naito Parkway South. Turn left at the light on Market Street / I-5 South sign. Turn left at first light onto Montgomery and take an immediate left onto Harbor Way. RiverPlace Hotel is located at the end of Harbor Way.

From I-5 (northbound), turn left to merge onto I-5 North toward Portland. Take exit 299B on the left for I-405 North toward US 26 W / City Center. Take exit

1A on the left toward Naito Parkway / Japanese-American Historical Plaza. Merge onto SW Harbor Drive. Turn right onto SW Montgomery Street. Take the first left onto SW Harbor Way. The hotel is at the end of the cul-de-sac.

Public transportation: The N-S line Portland streetcar makes stops at Meade, Gaines, Gibbs, and Lowell. The 35 and 36 buses serve the area. An overhead tram transports people to and from the campus at the top of Marquam Hill.

Overview: These urban parks are among the most recent additions to the system. The goals of both parks include providing residents of high-density buildings a pleasant outdoor experience, with places for individual quietude, neighborly conversation, and group events. South Waterfront Park is closely tied to the river, while Caruthers Park is near the Oregon Center for Health and Healing office building and serves several surrounding high-rises.

The Walk

▸Begin at the RiverPlace Hotel.

▸Turn toward the Willamette River and walk south, with the river on your left. Walk past the marina and some small shops and restaurants. Pass McCormick & Schmick's seafood restaurant. In summer this part of the walk is filled with outdoor diners.

▸Turn right on the corner by the restaurant where the waterfront path meets Montgomery Street. Cross Montgomery on the left side of the small traffic circle filled with flowers. The north end of South Waterfront Park is on

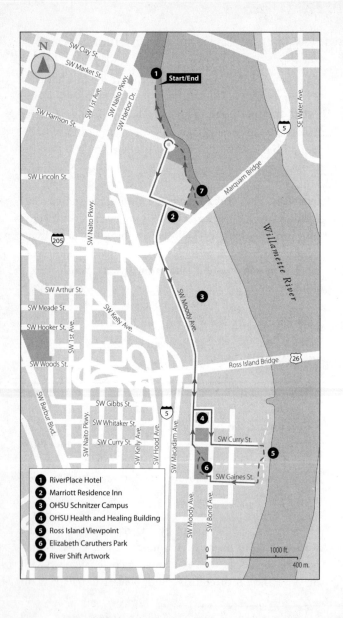

N

SW Clay St.
SW Market St.

1 Start/End

SW Harrison St.

SW 1st Ave.
SW Naito Pkwy.
SW Harbor Dr.

SW Lincoln St.

7

Marquam Bridge

SW Naito Pkwy.

2

Willamette River

205

SE Water Ave.

5

SW Arthur St.

SW Moody Ave.

3

SW Meade St.

SW Kelly Ave.

SW Hooker St.

SW 1st Ave.

SW Woods St.

Ross Island Bridge   26

U.S. 26

SW Barbur Blvd.

SW Gibbs St.

SW Naito Pkwy.

SW Whitaker St.

SW Kelly Ave.

SW Curry St.

SW Hood Ave.

SW Macadam Ave.

5

4

SW Curry St.

6

5

SW Gaines St.

1 RiverPlace Hotel
2 Marriott Residence Inn
3 OHSU Schnitzer Campus
4 OHSU Health and Healing Building
5 Ross Island Viewpoint
6 Elizabeth Caruthers Park
7 River Shift Artwork

SW Moody Ave.

SW Bond Ave.

0   1000 ft.
0   400 m.

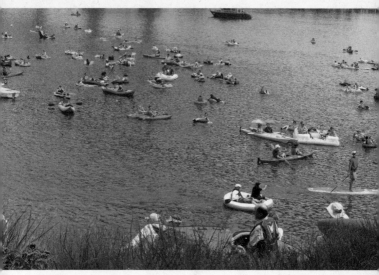

The annual Big Float celebrates the now-clean Willamette River. *Dick Lukins*

your left. Thick plantings provide private outdoor sitting spots next to small pools, and a slightly sunken courtyard protects you from the wind on breezy days.

▶Exit the park on River Drive between a small stone restaurant and the restroom building. Continue straight south on River Drive. Two large underground parking garages are on either side of the street, and one honors validated parking vouchers from some area restaurants and shops.

▶Stop at Moody/Harrison Street. You will see a streetcar stop on a traffic island straight ahead. Turn left on Harrison and go east toward the large redbrick Marriott Residence Inn.

▸Cross Moody by the hotel entrance. Take the sidewalk south alongside the Marriott, passing their parking garage.

▸Continue on Moody to the junction with Sheridan Street. Push the button at the traffic signal to cross Sheridan and continue south on the sidewalk. This sidewalk is well used by bikers, runners, and walkers. Watch for the arrows and signs on the pavement, as the sides for walkers and bikers switch every so often.

▸Pass the streetcar stop at Meade. Across Moody on the riverside is the Schnitzer campus for OHSU's new Collaborative Life Sciences Building, encouraging researchers from Portland State University and Oregon State University to work together on projects. There will also be a new dental school building, and after 2015 there will be access to a light rail and pedestrian/bicycle bridge.

▸Continue south under the Ross Island Bridge.

▸Stop at the streetcar plaza at Gibbs Street. On your right is the access to the Hooley Pedestrian Bridge west over the interstate highway.

▸On your left is the beginning of the aerial tram line. It goes straight up and overhead to the Marquam Campus of OHSU, the main site of the hospital on the top of "Pill Hill." The Veterans Hospital is also there. Turn left and cross Moody at the traffic signal.

►Turn left and continue along the north side of the OHSU Health and Wellness Building. If the building is open, you can access water and restrooms inside.

►Cross the streetcar tracks to the east side of Bond. The large blue cranes overhead on your left mark the Zidell Barge Company, the only survivor of the area's former industry. Zidell once dismantled decommissioned ships after World War II, and now builds steel barges for river traffic.

►Turn right to Whitaker. Turn left and go east one block to River Parkway. Cross River Parkway and turn right along the chain-link fence toward a large cluster of condo and apartment skyscrapers. This is the South Waterfront redevelopment area, a favorite setting for such television shows as *Leverage* and *Portlandia*. Once a brownfield polluted by industrial waste, the land has been capped, filled in, and raised to become a green walkable neighborhood with as few cars as possible. Building vertically allows maximum population in minimum space, while the varied street level is filled with small shops and open sitting areas.

►At Curry, turn left toward the river and continue to the end, past the off-leash dog park and the U-pick dahlia gardens.

►Cross Curry. Take the riverside walkway behind the buildings. Note the pole supporting the osprey nest. Ospreys have been nesting in this area for many years. Across the river is a great view of the north tip of Ross Island. Ross

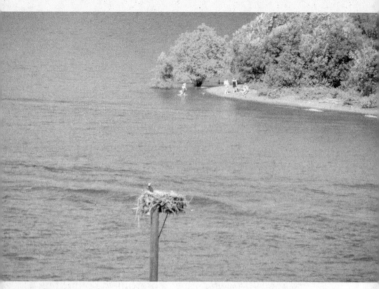

Osprey, eagles, and herons make their homes on these islands. *Dick Lukins*

is the main island of a four-island cluster. A levee at the southern end connects it to Hardtack Island on the east, forming a lagoon in the center where they mine gravel. Tiny East Island and Toe Island are to the south. Part of the island was given to the city as a natural area, since it is home to osprey, eagles, and herons. If you are sharp-eyed you may spot the heron rookery near the north end.

▶Continue on the brick path, enjoying the river traffic. Much is commercial, but almost every type of watercraft can be seen here, including the Portland Spirit dinner boat. You may see the dragon boats—large shells with a

dragonhead on the prow, raced in the June Rose Festival—
and in summer there are usually canoes and kayaks parked
along the shoreline on the island.

▶Take the walk to the end and then turn right on Gaines.
Take the sidewalk past Atwater Place apartments and go
one block to River Parkway. Cross, pass the John Ross condos' park-like plaza on your right, and continue to Bond.
Cross Bond and continue a few feet to a boardwalk. Turn
right into Elizabeth Caruthers Park.

This 2-acre neighborhood park was designed as a community space for a high-rise neighborhood, and to be as sustainable and natural as possible. Take the boardwalk into the
park between benches and the lawn. The raised bolts on the
boardwalk edges can be felt through the soles of shoes, warn-
ing pedestrians that they are close to low spots and swales.

At the southwest end of the park is the outdoor art
piece called *Song Cycles:* overhead spinning bicycle wheels
with clickers attached to catch the wind. They provide
background sounds for park users.

▶Turning right at the boardwalk "T," continue to the concrete walkway, and turn left. Follow it as it curves around
the back of the mound to the center of the park. The top of
the hill has a view between the buildings to the river beyond.

▶Continue to the path until you see a stack of timbers
on your left. Turn left on the rubbery surface into the
pool area where, in summer, little fountains spurt out of
stepping-stones. The stacked timber also serves as climbing
equipment and good sitting spots.

▶Pass by the pool to your right and exit on a sandy path. Turn left into another small sitting area almost hidden by the shrubs around it. A glossy stone table sits in the center of the benches, and a boulder on the west side marks the site of the first settlers' cabin. This is also where Elizabeth Caruthers and her son Finice took up their land claims after they arrived on the Oregon Trail from Tennessee. She was the first single woman to have her claim to land acknowledged by the US Supreme Court. Looking east from the stone benches, you can also see chairs and tables around the bocce court.

▶Exit the park on Curry and turn left to Moody. Turn right, cross Curry, and continue past a green lawn, which is the roof of OHSU's underground parking lot.

▶Cross Whitaker and pass the OHSU building to the crosswalk at Gibbs. Turn left, cross Gibbs, and turn right on the sidewalk you traversed earlier. Continue on this to the Sheridan Street traffic signal.

▶Push the signal to trigger the traffic light, and cross to the east side, under the Marquam Bridge.

▶Turn left and walk north. Continue alongside the Marriott Residence Inn service areas.

▶Turn right under the large arch that defines the hotel's front entrance. Then turn left and cross River Parkway into the South Waterfront Park. Eventually this walk will connect the South Waterfront Greenway with the Tom McCall Riverfront Park. Meanwhile, it is a lovely, quiet area for the

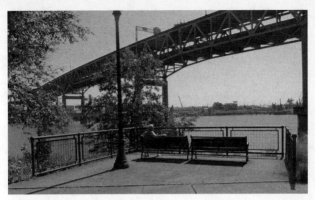

South Waterfront Park has access to the river.

many apartments to the west, and offers access to the river. It also offers river access for boats and rubber rafts.

▶Continue on the walk to the gravel path on your right. Go up the small slope to the river walkway. The basalt rocks on your right are part of Mathieu Gregoire's *River Shift,* showing various effects of the river on the land. Note the visible strata on some of the rocks.

▶Turn right to take the walkway south to the circle at its end under the bridge. More rocks are here at the circle. A path on the left by the riverside will take you down to the river.

▶Return up to the main path and retrace your steps to *River Shift.* Continue north. Pass another path offering river access.

▶Continue north. You will come to an area with paths, benches, and gardens.

▸Continue on the main path through the gardens until you see the traffic circle at Montgomery Street. If you are looking for public restrooms, turn left, cross, and turn left on Montgomery, then right onto River Walk. Pass some offices and you'll find a nice restroom building on your right.

▸Join the River Walk just ahead and follow it to your starting point at the RiverPlace Hotel.

SOUTHEAST

Walk 16: Eastbank Esplanade

📷 🏢 ♿

General location: Downtown Portland Waterfront, west of I-5

Special attractions: Willamette River waterfront

Difficulty: Easy, flat

Distance: 3 miles

Estimated time: 2 hours

Services: Restrooms, and there are water fountains in various locations.

Restrictions: Dogs must be leashed.

For more information: Contact the Portland Oregon Visitors Association, 701 Southwest 6th Avenue, Portland, OR 97204; (503) 275-8355; travelportland.com; or the RiverPlace Hotel, 1510 Southwest Harbor Way, Portland, OR 97201; (503) 228-3233; riverplacehotel.com.

Getting started: From I-5 (southbound), take the exit to City Center / OMSI. Take the right lane and follow signs to Morrison Street/Bridge. Stay in the right lane on Morrison Bridge. Take the Naito Parkway exit and loop onto Naito Parkway South. Turn left at the light on Market Street / I-5 South sign. Turn left at first light onto Montgomery and take an immediate left onto Harbor Way. RiverPlace Hotel is located at the end of Harbor Way.

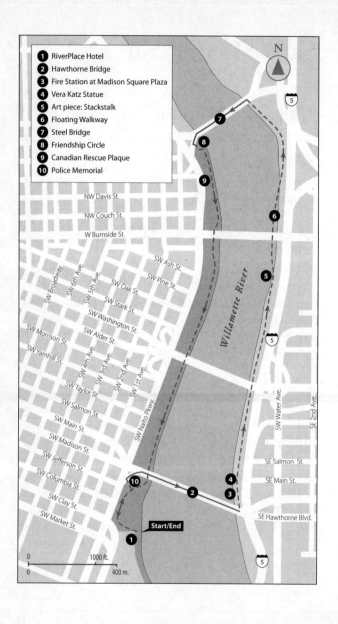

1 RiverPlace Hotel
2 Hawthorne Bridge
3 Fire Station at Madison Square Plaza
4 Vera Katz Statue
5 Art piece: Stackstalk
6 Floating Walkway
7 Steel Bridge
8 Friendship Circle
9 Canadian Rescue Plaque
10 Police Memorial

N

NW Davis St.
NW Couch St.
W Burnside St.

SW Ash St.
SW Oak St.
SW Pine St.
SW Stark St.
SW Washington St.
SW Alder St.

SW Broadway
SW 6th Ave.
SW 5th Ave.
SW Morrison St.
SW Yamhill St.
SW 4th Ave.
SW 3rd Ave.
SW 2nd Ave.
SW 1st Ave.
SW Taylor St.
SW Salmon St.
SW Main St.
SW Madison St.
SW Jefferson St.
SW Columbia St.
SW Clay St.
SW Market St.

SW Naito Pkwy.

Willamette River

SW Water Ave.
SE 2nd Ave.

SE Salmon St.
SE Main St.
SE Hawthorne Blvd.

Start/End

0   1000 ft.
0   400 m.

From I-5 (northbound), turn left to merge onto I-5 North toward Portland. Take exit 299B on the left for I-405 North toward US 26 W / City Center. Take exit 1A on the left toward Naito Parkway / Japanese-American Historical Plaza. Merge onto SW Harbor Drive. Turn right onto SW Montgomery Street. Take the first left onto SW Harbor Way. The hotel is at the end of the cul-de-sac. **Public transportation:** Bus 96 stops at Harbor Drive and Montgomery. The Portland Streetcar, N-S line, has stops at Harrison Street, and at Moody/River Drive. All stops are about a half mile from RiverPlace.

Overview: The addition of the Eastbank Esplanade means that a walker can loop Portland's east and west riverfronts from the Burnside Bridge to the Hawthorne Bridge, with a variety of interesting views. Both sides have displays on waterfront history.

The Walk

▸Start the walk at the RiverPlace Hotel. Take the path that curves around the grassy bowl on the riverside that often hosts musical events in nice weather.

▸Stop at the right of the circular flower bed and look for the brick wall across the grass on your left. This is the Police Memorial, a quiet circle honoring those who have given their lives to protect the community.

▸Go toward the memorial.

▸Take the path on the left toward the bike sign saying EASTBOUND. This is the ramp to the Hawthorne Bridge.

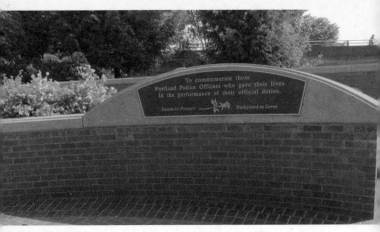

The Police Memorial offers a quiet place to reflect on lives lost.

Take this around and up to the bridge. Stay on this south side of the bridge until you reach the east bank of the Willamette River. This 1910 bridge is the nation's oldest operating vertical lift bridge, lifting for river traffic about eight times a day. The pedestrian/bicycle path is concrete, but the steel grating for highway traffic reduces bridge weight. As you get near the end of the bridge, look south to see the dock for racing sculls and kayaks.

▸Take the ramp on your right down to the Eastbank Esplanade near the dock.

▸Turn right on the path to the Madison Square Plaza in front of the Portland Fire Station. The landscape architects included many features along the way to help you understand what you see. Note the large map inscribed in the pavement by the fire station. It gives you a good idea of the reach of this 187-mile commercial waterway, which begins in the mountains to the south and joins the Columbia River at the north end.

A water fountain provides a cold drink of water. Scattered on the plaza around it are five specimens of columnar basalt. Although these look man-made, this type of basalt formed naturally on the vertical fractures that were created when flowing lava cooled quickly. The Columbia River Basin is one of the places where columnar basalts are found.

▶On your left is a ramp leading down to a dock used by fireboats. The walk/bike path is on the right of the station's fire engine bay. Go north on this path, with the river on your left. The esplanade is also a demonstration project for improved habitat areas and riverbank restoration. The replacement of riprap with bioengineered banks planted with native vegetation means that water runoff is captured and cleaned before entering the river.

▶As you head north you will find thirteen lampposts along your way, with attached street signs marking where city streets once met the river. Interpretive panels attached to the pole markers provide information about the bridges, river history, and the mile-long harbor wall seen on the west bank. This first one tells about Lewis and Clark.

Just south of the Main Street marker, the Bill Bane bronze sculpture of Vera Katz acts as a "meet-up" place for the bicyclists, walkers, and runners who share this path. Note the Portland rose on her lapel. She was the visionary mayor from 1992 to 2005 who helped bring the esplanade dream to fruition.

▶At Salmon Street, a display sign provides information about the river's history. Restrooms can be found under the highway bridge, and more parking is available east of those.

More information is on signs around the pillars at Taylor.

▶A copper sculpture, *Echo Gate,* is beneath the Morrison Bridge on the east side of the path. A reminder of the actual piers and Shanghai tunnels of Portland's past, it's the first of four pieces of public art that you'll see on the walk ahead created by a group of local artists. This is Portland's newest bascule bridge (drawbridge), built in 1958.

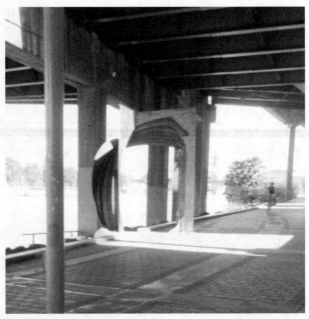

A local artist created *Echo Gate.*

▶At Alder Street a public fishing pier confirms how the river has been cleaned up. Now it's home to beavers, ducks, geese, herons, steelhead, and salmon—and fishermen.

▶On the right of a cantilevered walkway is a mossy concrete seawall, a remnant of early maritime shipping. At this south end is a metal lantern with hundreds of prismatic pieces of art glass. Entitled *Ghost Ship*, it pays homage to the many ships that went down in crossing the Columbia River bar, as well as those that came safely through Portland.

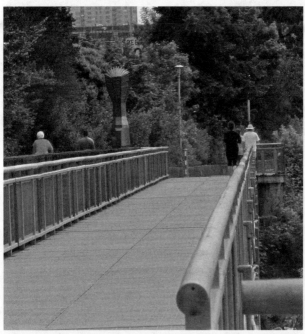

The *Ghost Ship* sculpture pays homage to the ships crossing the Columbia River bar.

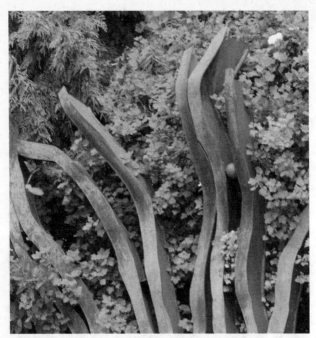

Can you find the child's ball embedded in this *Alluvial Wall* art piece?

▶At the far end of the seawall is *Stackstalk,* a "hybrid beacon, part masthead, part wheat stem, part smokestack" made of rolled steel tubes supporting a glass fishing float at the top. Just beyond, the final art piece, entitled *Alluvial Wall,* clings to a concrete retaining wall. Resembling what you might see on a beach after the tide goes out, it alludes to the "interwoven layers of the river's preindustrial geology and human artifacts." Many black metal objects are embedded among the copper kelp-like strips, ranging from a railroad spike, a morel mushroom, and a child's ball. What can you find?

From here you can see you're nearing the 1926 Burnside Bridge—a bascule bridge (drawbridge) like the Morrison. Ahead of you, tall red pilings capped with white cones mark the floating walkway, constructed because highways above did not leave enough shoreline for a path. At 1,200 feet, it's the longest floating walkway of its kind in the United States, and the only bridge on this river designed by a woman engineer.

▸Don't take the path leading to a flight of steps going up to the bridge exiting on North Burnside; instead, take the ramp to your left and the floating walkway. The concrete underfoot makes it feel solid, but you can also feel motion caused by fluctuating river tides.

▸At the far end is the Kevin J. Duckworth Memorial Dock, named for one of the city's former Blazer basketball players. This public boat dock provides moorage for recreational

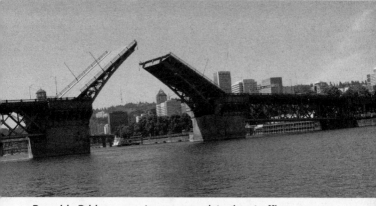

Burnside Bridge opens to accommodate river traffic.

boaters as well as space for future commercial uses. Take time to read the display sign about the "scow" villages that once inhabited this area, predecessors of the houseboat villages still clustered on the Willamette at different sites.

▸At the end of the walkway, turn left and enter the River Walk on the bottom level of the 1912 Steel Bridge. This is the only double-deck vertical lift bridge of its kind in the world. According to *The Portland Bridge Book,* the lower deck (built for trains) may be lifted independently, telescoping into trusses of the upper deck (built for street railways, pedestrians and bicyclists, and vehicles) to move out of the way of river traffic.

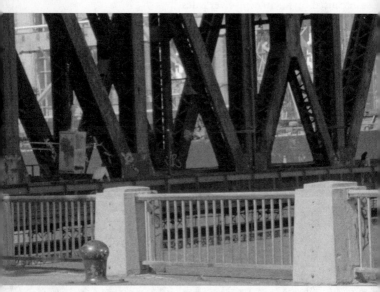

All manner of vehicles as well as pedestrians share the Steel Bridge.

▶The train-level bike/pedestrian path, about 30 feet above the Willamette River, was cantilevered off the bottom deck in 1991. It's held in place by pilings sunk into a huge concrete base and only "kisses" the bridge, adding no weight to the bridge itself. It offers pedestrians and bicyclists a route across the river and provides a stunning overlook from which to view the downtown cityscape.

▶Exit the Steel Bridge at the north end of Tom McCall Waterfront Park. You will find yourself at the Friendship Circle, created to commemorate thirty years of sister-city relations with Sapporo, Japan. Lee Kelly and Michael Stirling designed the 20-foot-tall stainless towers in the center, which periodically emit (electronically) the sounds of ancient Japanese instruments. One hundred ornamental cherry trees surround the circle and line the walkway south.

▶Continue south on the river walkway. From here, you are repeating some of the waterfront walk in this book's Walk 1: Riverfront and Old Town.

▶Where you see steps coming down from Everett Street, look for the boulder at the north end of their base. The brass plaque on it honors the Canadian embassy in Iran. When the Iranians overthrew the Shah, they captured the American embassy and imprisoned all the workers inside for 444 days. Several diplomats who managed to flee were eventually hidden in the Canadian embassy, at great risk to the Canadian ambassador. This is a thank-you for what became known as the "Canadian Caper," dramatized in the Oscar-nominated 2012 film *Argo*.

▶Watch out for fat steel mooring posts called "bollards." They are used for the permanent mooring of the *Portland,* a maritime museum up ahead, and for the navy ships which sail in each year for the Rose Festival.

▶Keep going south under the Burnside Bridge. This is the site of the Saturday Market, well known for its wide variety of crafts and food.

▶Continue on the walkway until you come to a stone path leading to the right. Take this into the Japanese-American Historical Plaza, a reminder of the days when American citizens of Japanese origin were forced to leave their homes for relocation camps.

▶Two bronze cylinders, *Songs of Innocence* and *Songs of Experience,* carved with sketches of soldiers and civilians, are the centerpieces here. Fractured pavement in the center of the plaza represents the internees' broken dreams. Verses in both Japanese and English by three noted Oregon poets are inscribed on thirteen basalt and granite pillars. The last stone includes a reminder of how the forced internment of Japanese Americans during World War II violated every single article of the US Constitution and the Bill of Rights. It displays excerpts from the Civil Liberties Act of 1988, and the official apology by the US Congress for the unlawful imprisonment of US citizens.

▶Turn right on the walkway when you leave the Japanese-American Historical Plaza. Enjoy the view of Portland's skyline, but remember the bicyclists, runners, and skateboarders who also enjoy this river walk.

▸Walk by the polished, stainless-steel *Sculpture Stage,* and enter the square with the Bill Naito Legacy Fountain. Many of Portland's outdoor activities and festivals take place here. The wide sitting steps "remember Bill Naito as a businessman and true citizen, son of this Old Town neighborhood, a tireless champion of the preservation of its history and for the potential of its people." The former Front Street was renamed Naito Parkway in his honor.

▸Continue walking south. The ship moored on your left is the *Portland,* the last steam-powered sternwheel tugboat built in the United States in 1947. Though the tug pilots prized the sternwheelers for their unique ship-handling ability, diesels finally took over. This ship has been restored by charitable grants and thousands of hours of volunteer work. It doubled as the *Lauren Belle* in the 1994 movie, *Maverick,* and now has a new role as the Oregon Maritime Museum. It contains many artifacts from Portland's rich seafaring history, and is open to the public. Check the museum website for the current schedules. An old navy barge, the *Russell,* is docked in front of the *Portland,* and serves as a workspace for the volunteers.

Look for the smokestack on the far right of the walkway. This is from the battleship USS *Oregon,* which saw action in Cuba during the 1898 Spanish-American War. A bicentennial time capsule inside the stack is to be opened in 2076.

As you walk along, you'll see many signs pointing out sites of early Portland history. Not too far from the Portland is a sign marking "The Clearing," which Massachusetts captain John Couch thought "a good spot for a seaport." Other signs mark "Indian Camps, 1845," the first wharf built in 1846, and a Stephens family's land claim across the river. The next marker designates the 1845 townsite. The Lownsdale land-claim marker is at Morrison Street. This 1887 Morrison Bridge was the first of three bridges built over the Willamette River.

▶Continue to the Salmon Street Springs fountains. The fountain near Naito Parkway is a child's delight, with a variety of three spray patterns (bollards, wedding cake, and misters) that seem to change constantly. Steps along the riverside provide a place to sit, admire the river, or wait your turn for a warm-weather river cruise on the *Portland Spirit*.

▶Follow the walkway under the Hawthorne Bridge. Across the river is the redbrick tower at OMSI—the Oregon Museum of Science and Industry.

▶Signs at the plaza here tell about the Willamette River cleanup under former governor Tom McCall's leadership. They also explain how a six-lane expressway was torn down in 1974 to create this park.

▶Turn west from here and go up the path toward the Police Memorial. Take time to look at the inscriptions, names, and dates on the walls before continuing back to your starting point at the RiverPlace Hotel.

Walk 17: Eastmoreland, Crystal Springs, and Reed College

📷 ✕ 🏢 ♿

General location: Southeast Portland, 5 miles east of downtown and 12 miles south of the airport

Special attractions: A classic neighborhood, photogenic small college campus, and rhododendron gardens surrounding a spring-fed lake

Difficulty: Easy; mostly flat, on sidewalks, and the main walk is wheelchair-accessible

Distance: About 2.5 miles

Estimated time: 1.5 hours, plus optional time spent enjoying the Rhododendron Garden

Services: Restrooms and water are available at Reed College and Crystal Springs Rhododendron Garden.

Restrictions: Crystal Springs is open April 1 to September 30 from 6 a.m. to 10 p.m., and October 1 to March 31 from 6 a.m. to 6 p.m. No entrance fee from Labor Day through February. A $3 admission fee is charged between 10 a.m. and 6 p.m., Thursday through Monday, March through Labor Day; free for children under twelve. For information on Reed College events, check its website http://reedevents.reed.edu/reed_events.html.

For more information: Contact Portland Parks and Recreation, or Friends of the Crystal Springs Rhododendron Garden.

Getting started: Reed College is in southeast Portland. From I-205 go to the Foster Road exit, turn west to 82nd

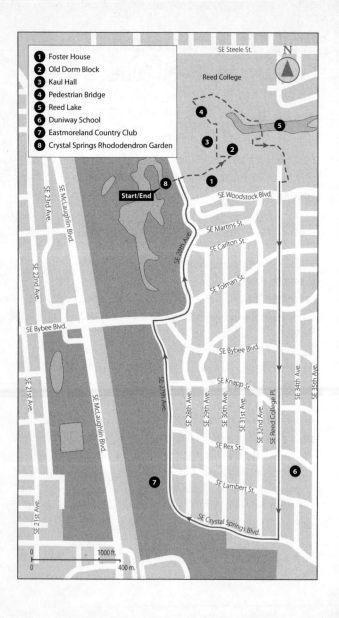

1 Foster House
2 Old Dorm Block
3 Kaul Hall
4 Pedestrian Bridge
5 Reed Lake
6 Duniway School
7 Eastmoreland Country Club
8 Crystal Springs Rhododendron Garden

SE Steele St.

Reed College

N

Start/End

SE Woodstock Blvd.

SE Martins St.

SE Carlton St.

SE 28th Ave.

SE Tolman St.

SE McLaughlin Blvd.

SE 23rd Ave.

SE 22nd Ave.

SE Bybee Blvd.

SE Bybee Blvd.

SE Knapp St.

SE 21st Ave.

SE McLaughlin Blvd.

SE 27th Ave.

SE 28th Ave.

SE 29th Ave.

SE 30th Ave.

SE 31st Ave.

SE 32nd Ave.

SE Reed College Pl.

SE 34th Ave.

SE 35th Ave.

SE Rex St.

SE Lambert St.

SE Crystal Springs Blvd.

SE 21st Ave.

0   1000 ft.
0   400 m.

Avenue, south on 82nd, and turn right on Woodstock Boulevard just past the 39th Avenue intersection.

Public transportation: From downtown, take Bus 19 (Woodstock) which stops at two Reed College stations on the north side of Woodstock: one at 39th and one at 36th. Contact TriMet for information about fares and schedules (trimet.org).

Overview: The original Crystal Springs Farm became the lovely neighborhoods of Eastmoreland and Westmoreland. Part of the farm was donated in 1909 to found Reed College. At the time, it was pastureland with few trees; most of the century-old trees now gracing the campus were collected from other Oregon regions by W. F. Eliot. The American Rhododendron Society established a nearby test garden for rhododendrons and azaleas, which became part of the Portland Parks System in 1950. You will walk by the extensive Eastmoreland Golf Club, the Rhododendron Garden, and through the campus of Reed College.

The Walk

▶The walk begins at the Reed College west parking entrance on SE 28th Avenue, across from the Crystal Springs Rhododendron Garden. This is a classically beautiful campus, with many redbrick buildings designed by noted Portland architect, A. E. Doyle. The Tudor Gothic design is reminiscent of old English manor halls.

▶Start at the large campus map sign on the campus side of the parking lot near the emergency information post.

▶Take the walkway on the right. Pass a beautiful large chain tree as you walk past Foster House (a residence hall) to the "Y."

▶Angle left at the "Y," passing the McNaughten residence hall, and then take the diagonal walk across the Great Lawn to the Old Dorm Block. This 1912 A. E. Doyle residence hall is still prized student housing, with fireplaces in nearly every room. The building is studded with "grotesques"—gargoyle-like heads never intended to spout water. Two are on either side of the large "sally port" in the center of the building: *Lux* grins at the day while *Nox* closes his eyes.

▶Turn left on the sidewalk back to the walkway by the Anna Mann residence hall. Turn right, passing the lawn in front of the Performing Arts Center before reaching Kaul Hall. This center is used for many musical events. The Gray Campus Center is on your right. The west end

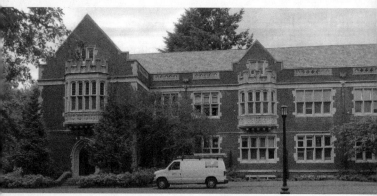

The Old Dorm is still considered desirable real estate.

of the building houses the Commons dining rooms, and is attached to the original A. E. Doyle student center on the east end. Water, snacks, and restrooms are here.

▸Stay on the walk between Kaul and Gray until you see a stop sign at Botsford Drive. Cross the roadway diagonally to the pedestrian bridge.

▸Take the bridge across the canyon. Dense foliage may prevent a view of the stream far below, but you can clearly hear it burbling over the rocks.

▸This north canyon area has sports facilities and many residence halls. Turn right on the paved sidewalk by the tennis courts. The walkway splits three ways. On your right a gravel trail goes down the canyon and around the perimeter of Reed Lake. Take the center walkway behind Griffin and stay right of the residence halls skirting the north side of the lake.

▸Take Canyon Bridge south over crystal-clear Reed Lake. Ahead is Eliot Hall, one of the original campus buildings. Take the walk to your right around the building to the door at the southwest corner. Before entering, note the campus seal over the door. The griffin came from founder Simeon Reed's family crest, and is now the mascot for the college. If you go through this door, you can visit the lovely English chapel with its many details copied from tenth-century chapels. Outside on your right is an impressive sculpture by Portland's notable Lee Kelly, who was a visiting professor here.

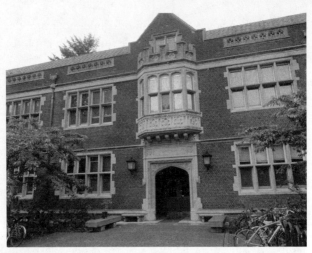
Eliot Hall is one of the original Reed College buildings.

▶Take the walkway on the east side of the library, between the library and science buildings. Here is another Lee Kelly sculpture, this one made from Cor-Ten steel, and very different from the other.

▶Proceed south to the road, turn right to the traffic circle, and then go south past the Reed College pillar, to the main entrance on Woodstock Boulevard.

▶Cross Woodstock to the east side of Reed College Place.

▶Go south on this street. Note the well-preserved old elms in the center parkway. These are survivors of the Dutch elm epidemic that decimated trees throughout the United States. This well-maintained college neighborhood has a traditional feel.

Note the houses on either side of the parkway. The varied architecture reflects the times in which they were built. These are unostentatious family houses rather than showplaces, blending individual designs into a picture-perfect and child-friendly neighborhood. Meticulous landscaping adds to the ambience.

▶Cross Tolman Street and walk four blocks to Rex Street, passing Claybourne, Bybee, and Knapp.

The classically designed school on the corner of Rex and Reed College Place was named for Abigail Scott Duniway, an early Oregon leader of the women's rights movement. Lawns, since replaced by blacktop play and parking areas, once surrounded the school.

▶Cross Rex Street and then cross Reed College Place. Continue south on the west side past Lambert Street, and go one

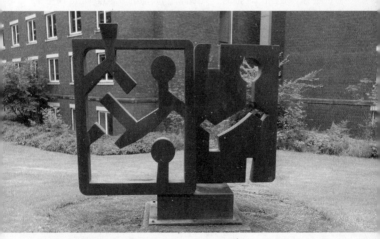

Lee Kelly designed many Portland fountains.

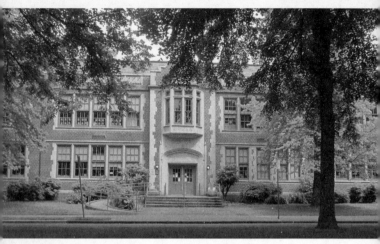

The Duniway School was designed by A. E. Doyle.

more block to Crystal Springs Road. Follow the sidewalk around to the west as it turns right. On the far side of this road you can see the swings of the neighborhood play park.

▶Continue along this sidewalk, passing streets from 32nd until you reach 27th. At 27th the road curves to the north. You can see the Eastmoreland Country Club on your left across 27th. More lovely homes line this street.

▶Keep going north on the east side of 27th until you reach SE Bybee Boulevard. The parking areas for the golf course are across the street. A small park is on your right.

▶Cross Bybee with care, as there are no stop signs here. The sidewalk and your route turn east, skirting the edge of the golf course.

▶At the intersection of Woodstock and SE 28th, the golf course comes to an end. Continue north on the west sidewalk along SE 28th to the Crystal Springs Rhododendron Garden. It is definitely worth a visit at any time of the year. The springs that gave the area its name still come out from rock walls and bubble up to form numerous ponds, including the college's Reed Lake. The gardens are home to many birds and plants besides the spectacular spring-blooming rhododendrons: camellias, dove trees, and a variety of ferns and water irises.

▶If you prefer to return directly to your starting point, take the crosswalk at Woodstock and 28th. Stay on the east side of 28th and return to the starting point at the Reed College west parking entrance.

Walk 18: Mount Tabor Park

General location: The east side of Portland, south of I-84 and east of I-5

Special attractions: Walk on top of the only extinct volcano cinder cone in the center of a US city. There are natural areas, reservoirs, and views of Portland. All streets here are labeled SE.

Difficulty: Moderate, with one hill, entirely on paved roads; although the walk is suitable for strollers, it is quite steep, and many areas are not accessible to wheelchairs.

Distance: 2 miles

Estimated time: 1 hour

Services: Restrooms and water can be found at the information center and at the summit. Also available are a picnic shelter; playground; and basketball, volleyball, and tennis courts.

Restrictions: Portland enforces its scoop law. Dogs must be leashed to and from the off-leash areas, and their droppings must be disposed of. Note: The park is completely closed to cars on Wednesdays. This makes the road from the summit a favorite for skateboarders, so watch out.

For more information: Contact Portland Parks and Recreation.

Getting started: From I-84 eastbound, take exit 5, OR 213 (82nd Avenue), south to SE Stark Street. Go right (west) on Stark, following the signs to Mount Tabor. When you reach SE 69th Avenue, go left (south) straight into the park, and turn right on the first road. There is a sign for pedestrians regarding a flight of steps that leads up into the park. If you are walking into the park from the bus stop, you can take a flight of steps up to Taylor Street and walk to the parking area.

Public transportation: Bus 15 (Mount Tabor) stops at SE 69th Avenue and Yamhill Street. Contact TriMet for information about fares and schedules (trimet.org).

Overview: Plympton Kelly, an early settler in this neighborhood, named this hill "Mount Tabor" after he read about a battle fought by the French against the Muslims near Mount Tabor in Palestine. Not until 1912, many years after the hill was developed into a neighborhood park, was it discovered to be an extinct volcano. The summit is 600 feet above the surrounding area.

Paved roads, good views, and many dirt jogging paths make this a popular park with walkers, bicyclists, and runners. Many flights of steps throughout the park help people climb the steep slopes. A reporter for *The Oregonian* once counted 257 steps in all!

The three small pools are actually some of Portland's reservoirs, completed in 1894. Their stonework and castle-like buildings punctuate the park's natural beauty.

If the park roads are gated, park your car near the SE Yamhill & SE 69th entrance. Turn right on the paved Taylor Drive, and go west to the junction with SE North Tabor Drive.

Otherwise, park at the lot located at the junction of Taylor Drive and SE North Tabor Drive. You will find restrooms, a park welcome office, and an information board with park maps and information.

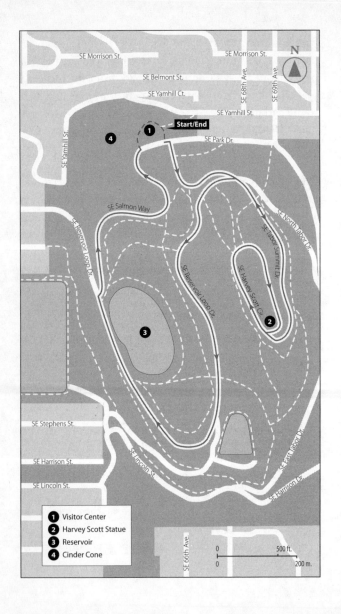

The Walk

▶Start here at the information board and walk south on North Tabor Drive, passing a playground and climbing the hill to a junction with Summit Drive. Walk through a small parking area and take the right gated road up a hill. This road is steep, but you will see many bicyclists and people pushing strollers up the hill. It is occasionally open to cars. Since it is winding, bicyclists and skateboarders cannot always see you, so be sure to keep to the left side.

▶You will come to two sets of stairs: One goes up the hill to your right, and the other goes down the hill to your left. A tennis court lies far below the road on your left. Ferns, wildflowers, and the leathery salal bushes hug the bank on your right.

▶Pass the stairs and follow the paved road as it curves around to the top of Mount Tabor.

▶Look for the stone steps just beyond the wide area at the crest. Take these up to the statue of Harvey Scott that crowns the grassy summit above the road. He was an influential newspaper editor and historian who adamantly opposed the woman's suffrage movement promoted by his sister, Abigail Scott Duniway.

▶Go down the steps under Scott's hand pointing to the west. There is a small bench here, and you will find others as you proceed to your right on the road around the Harvey Scott Circle.

You will get many glimpses of Portland through gaps in the trees. A great view of the city is near the north end of the circle. The charming building on the north side of the road resembling a small French cottage is actually a former restroom building. Vandalism has unfortunately forced its closure.

Lovely old Douglas firs crown the summit of Mount Tabor. As you stroll across this knoll, look for an official City of Portland survey benchmark in the ground near the far end of the knoll. A nearby bench is inscribed with the words TAKE TIME TO RELAX AND WATCH THE WORLD AROUND YOU.

▶Diagonally across from the bench are three flights of steps going down the hill. These lead back to the road near

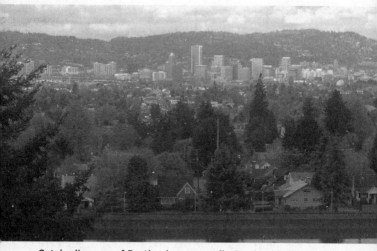

Catch glimpses of Portland as you walk. *Portland Parks & Recreation, Portland, OR*

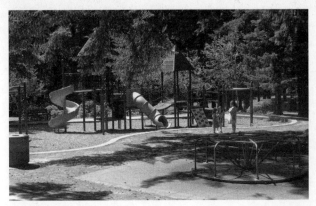

Children enjoy Mount Tabor Park's playground. *Portland Parks & Recreation, Portland, OR*

the playground. You can take these steps down or continue on the paved road back to the statue to retrace your path down the hill.

▶At the bottom of the hill, continue across the small parking area where the roads meet. You have gone about 1 mile and can easily return to your car from here.

▶If you wish to see more of the park, go left (west) around the barrier and follow Reservoir Loop Drive. This is a favorite road for dog and stroller walking, since only park vehicles are allowed here.

▶The road winds downhill. You can hear birdsong over the noise of distant traffic. A soapbox derby track is down the hill on your right, and you can see a large reservoir on the far side of the track. Continue past the trail leading off to the left, and you will see a smaller reservoir on your left.

▶Ignore another trail and a service road going off to the left. Keep on the main road around the hill—known as Poison Oak Hill—until you reach the large reservoir.

▶Follow the road along the tall fence on the west side of this reservoir. Notice the stone buildings that house machinery. You can see the soapbox derby track on the far side of the reservoir, while another reservoir lies down the hill on your left. Ahead are black iron gates.

▶Go through these gates. Take the road on the right, going uphill. Continue up this curving road, with two-way vehicular traffic. Walk on the left side of the road and listen carefully, since you cannot always see cars coming down the hill.

▶Pass a gravel trail with white bollards on your left and two small dirt trails on your right. Stay on the road and continue up "Picnic Hill" until you see the roof of the picnic shelter. A basketball court and amphitheater are on your left.

Just ahead you will see large lava boulders identifying the location of the throat of the volcano. You can read the sign telling about the eroded volcanic throat while viewing it on the hillside across from you.

▶After reading the sign, continue to your right to your starting point in the parking lot.

The roads in this park are unmarked, but as one mother pushing a baby carriage said, "It looks as if you can get lost, but you really can't. All the roads curve back to the starting point."

NORTHEAST

Walk 19: Convention Center and Lloyd Center

✕ 🛒 👫 🏢 ♿

General location: Northeast Portland, just east of I-5

Special attractions: The Oregon Convention Center, the Rose Garden and Coliseum sports arenas, the Lloyd Center Mall, and the Broadway shopping district

Difficulty: Easy, flat; entirely on paved sidewalk with curb cuts

Distance: 4 miles

Estimated time: 2 hours

Services: Wheelchair-accessible restrooms can be found in the Lloyd Center, the Convention Center, and the State Office Building. You will pass many restaurants and stores on this walk.

Restrictions: The Lloyd Center Mall is open weekdays from 10 a.m. to 9 p.m. and Sunday from 11 a.m. to 6 p.m. The Convention Center, Coliseum, and Rose Garden hours vary. Dogs must be leashed and their droppings picked up.

For more information: Contact the Portland Oregon Visitors Association or the Lloyd Center Mall.

Getting started: This walk starts at the Lloyd Center, at the intersection of Multnomah Street and 9th Avenue.

From I-5, take exit 302A / Convention Center, and turn onto eastbound Weidler Street. Follow the signs to Lloyd Center. At 9th Avenue, turn right and park at Lloyd Center. Parking garages and lots are situated at all four corners of the large mall: Halsey and 9th, Halsey and 15th, Multnomah and 9th, and Multnomah and 15th.

Public transportation: The MAX light-rail and the Portland Streetcar (CL line) run frequently between downtown Pioneer Place, Lloyd Center, and the Oregon Convention Center. The trains for Lloyd Center leave on the Yamhill Street side of Pioneer Place.

Overview: This busy convention and shopping district is easily reached by car, light-rail, bus, or streetcar.

The Walk

▸Begin this walk on the Lloyd Center plaza at the corner of Multnomah Street and 9th Avenue. Larry Kirkland's statue *Capitalism* is centered in a large pool in front of the Nordstrom department store entrance. A classical Ionic capital sits atop a column of fifty coins, with each coin having a funny or serious quotation about money along the edge. The winner of the art competition when the mall was renovated, it is an appropriate reminder of the relationship of money to a marketplace.

▸Walk east past Stanford's on the Multnomah Street side of Lloyd Center. Pass the Macy's department store entrance, and continue to the covered parking lot at the southeast corner of the building.

Several other winning art pieces were installed in the center. Six mailbox-like objects stand on concrete curbs

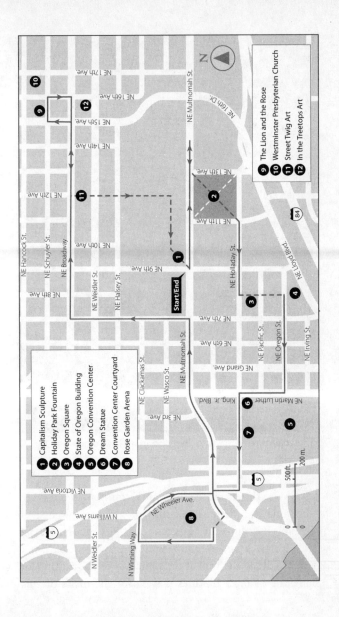

Legend:

1. Capitalism Sculpture
2. Holiday Park Fountain
3. Oregon Square
4. State of Oregon Building
5. Oregon Convention Center
6. Dream Statue
7. Convention Center Courtyard
8. Rose Garden Arena

9. The Lion and the Rose
10. Westminster Presbyterian Church
11. Street Twig Art
12. In the Treetops Art

Start/End

N

NE Victoria Ave.
NE 8th Ave.
NE Harcock St.
NE Schuyler St.
NE Broadway
NE 12th Ave.
NE 14th Ave.
NE 15th Ave.
NE 16th Ave.
NE 17th Ave.
NE 10th Ave.
NE 9th Ave.
NE Weidler St.
NE Halsey St.
NE Multnomah St.
NE 11th Ave.
NE 13th Ave.
NE 16th Dr.
NE Clackamas St.
NE Wasco St.
NE Multnomah St.
NE 7th Ave.
NE Holladay St.
NE 6th Ave.
NE Pacific St.
NE Oregon St.
NE Grand Ave.
NE Martin Luther King, Jr. Blvd.
NE Irving St.
NE Loyd Blvd.
84
NE 3rd Ave.
N Williams Ave.
N Winning Way
NE Wheeler Ave.
N Weidler St.
5
5
5

500 ft.
200 m.
0
0

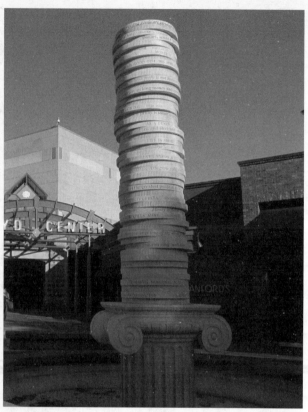

The sculpture reminds us that spending is a foundation for *Capitalism*.

just inside the entrance. These are *Consumer Reliquaries* by Christine Bourdette. Look through the window in each box to view different aspects of a 1980s shopping experience. *Free Flow*, a bronze sculpture by Al Goldsby, is situated along the wall at the right end of the parking lot. It is one of the sculptures created for the mall's original opening. Originally a two-tiered waterfall, it was redesigned as a river to fit this new location.

▸Exit on Multnomah Street and find the mosaic figure in the sidewalk. Artist Bill Will used a variety of materials in this *Sidewalk Robot*.

▸Turn right and retrace your steps to the signal by the Macy's entrance. Cross Multnomah Street at NE 13th into Holladay Park.

Ben Holladay gave this park to the city in 1870, before he lost all his money. This early railroad entrepreneur was known to many as "a sharpster, a con man, and a rake . . . wholly destitute of fixed principles of honesty, morality, or common decency." The park was renovated in 2000, with the earlier center fountain replaced by a spouting one—a delightful play place for children. Ted Savinar's *Constellation* has three separate freestanding bronze sculptures symbolizing the relationship between public and neighborhood gardens. The first is of an actual neighborhood gardener, another is a vase of cut flowers, and the third is an abstract molecule with its atoms made up of common household objects chosen by the neighbors in "Sullivan's Gulch," a former name for the district.

▸Go to Holladay Street, where there are stops for MAX light-rail and the Vintage Trolley. Turn right onto Holladay and walk to 9th. There is a drinking fountain on the northeast corner.

▸Cross 9th and then cross Holladay. Turn right and walk west to mid-block. This block is now the Oregon Square.

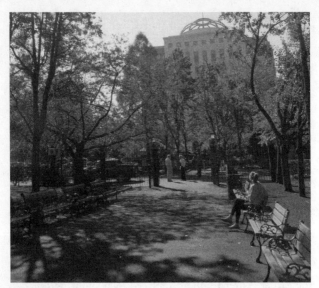

Oregon Square provides a restful approach to the State of
Oregon building.

The canopy over a large circle on your left provides cover
for the year-round Farmers' Market. Note the decorative
scarlet tulips around the perimeter, which catch water from
the canopy downspouts. A restroom building is located to
the south.

▶Turn south on the center walkway, and cross Pacific. The
impressive State of Oregon building is straight ahead.

▶Cross Oregon Street and enter the lobby. Look overhead
to see Don Merkt's mixed-media interpretation of the
Oregon state motto, "She Flies with Her Own Wings."
Large glass murals on the walls ahead illustrate legends

about Multnomah Falls and the Bridge of the Gods. The information desk has handouts about these stories.

▶Leave the lobby and turn left on Oregon Street going to NE 7th Avenue, passing a metered parking lot for visitors. On the corner is an interesting bronze called *Ideals*. Look inside these classically designed flowing robes and draped hood to see . . . emptiness.

▶Cross 7th Avenue at the crosswalk. The large building straight ahead is the Oregon Convention Center.

▶Staying on Oregon Street, walk two blocks to Grand Avenue crossing at the traffic signal. On your right is the Center Plaza. This serves as an annex to the Convention Center, as well as an outdoor exhibit hall, a place for outdoor entertainment, or simply a spot to enjoy a book in the sunshine.

▶Cross Martin Luther King Jr. Boulevard into the entrance courtyard of the Convention Center. If the center is open, take time to pick up the "Art & Fact Guide" brochure from the information desk and wander around to see the different pieces displayed in the lobby and restrooms. If the center is closed, you can still see some of it by peering through the glass doors. A dragon boat donated by Portland's sister city, Kaohsiung, Taiwan, hangs in the distance under the south green glass tower. This is the same type of boat you might see on the Willamette River when rowers are practicing for Rose Festival races. Under the north tower is *Principia*, a bronze Foucault pendulum that swings over a halo of gilded rays and a blue, inlaid terrazzo floor.

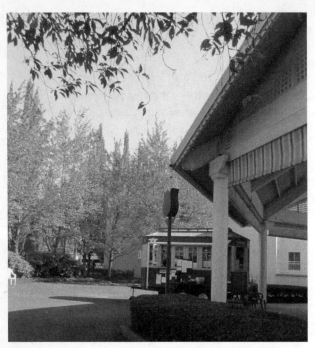
Note the downspouts camouflaged as decorative tulips.

▶Exit on Martin Luther King Jr. Boulevard and go left toward the MAX line. Michael Dente's *The Dream* statue is appropriately located at the corner of Martin Luther King Jr. Boulevard and Holladay Street.

▶Turn left here into the center's outdoor plaza, dominated by *Bell Circles II*. This "sound garden" was designed by Robert Coburn and incorporates two bronze bells in wooden bell houses. These were given by the Republic of China, and two of Portland's sister cities. They are rung electronically in a sequence designed by Coburn, "orienting the listener to time and space while expressing the link between Oregon and the Pacific Rim."

▸Turn back to Holladay Street. What looks like a landscape planting in front of you is actually an art piece, *Host Analog*. Artist Buster Simpson sawed a large Douglas fir into pieces and arranged them to resemble a broken Roman column. A watering system was installed, seeds and seedlings were planted in the segments, and the column became a typical Oregon "nurse log." The explanatory sign includes pictures showing how the piece looked when it was installed in 1991, so you can see how it has grown and changed in the interim.

▸Turn left and walk to 1st Avenue.

▸Cross Holladay and 1st Avenue at the signal and go under I-5. The trolley garage is here on the north side. A large window displays an original Lloyd Center trolley car.

▸Continue to your right around this building to Wheeler Street. A sign on this side of the building tells about the efforts of Dr. Lawrence Griffith and other volunteers in reactivating the rail system and trolley service.

▸Continue north to Multnomah and turn left. Cross Wheeler and walk half a block. A sculpture resembling the *Statue of Liberty*'s fallen crown is on the traffic median to your left. This is one of three pieces by Ilan Averbuch placed near the three entrances to the rose garden. They represent aspects of Antoine de Saint-Exupéry's *The Little Prince*.

▸Take the crosswalk into the Rose Quarter Plaza and go to the circular Rose Garden Arena, home of the NBA Portland Trail Blazers basketball team.

Ahead is a large square with two stone columns. This art piece is titled *Essential Elements*. Quiet during the day, flames leap up from the columns during night games, while jets of water spurt up and down in a random pattern.

▸Keep going right on the walkway around the building and to the center walkway. Memorial Coliseum, home to the Portland Winterhawks hockey team, is on your left.

▸The walkway ends at a short street, Winning Way. Across the way is a large bronze wing on a grassy knoll in front of the Madrona Studios. This is another *Little Prince* sculpture.

▸Walk right, past the Rose Garden Arena, back to the signal at Multnomah and Wheeler Streets. Turn left. Cross Wheeler at the light and keep on the left (north) side of Multnomah for four blocks, to Grand Avenue.

▸Cross Grand. You can see signs for the Lloyd Center. Continue straight for two more blocks, to 7th Avenue.

▸Cross 7th and turn left. Continue north for four street crossings to Broadway. Cross Broadway and turn right on Broadway. This street has many small interesting shops and restaurants.

▸Meander east along the north side of Broadway to 15th Avenue. Turn left, and proceed to Schuyler Street. Across from you on the corner is the 1905 Gustav Freiwald House, a charming Queen Anne–style home that is now The Lion and the Rose, a bed-and-breakfast. This is a remnant of the old Irvington district. Many similar houses were torn down or remodeled into apartments. Old trees provide welcome shade in the summer.

▶Turn right on Schuyler. Continue to 16th Avenue and cross to take a look at Westminster Presbyterian. Children's author Beverly Cleary once attended this stone church. She used it as the setting for the Christmas pageant in which character Ramona Quimby played a sheep.

The sanctuary contains seventy-two handworked needlepoint pew cushions reflecting the stained-glass windows. If you wish to admire these, continue north to Hancock Street and turn right to the office entrance at 1624 Hancock Street. Otherwise, turn right on 16th and go two blocks to Weidler. The large aluminum *Street Twig* at this corner represents the big-leaf maples common in this Sullivan Gulch neighborhood.

▶Return one block north to Broadway, turn left, and continue on the south side of Broadway, passing restaurants and shops.

▶Turn left at 12th Avenue. This is a walkway to the Lloyd Center. On the corner is a bright red sculpture, *In the Tree Tops,* by Margarita Leon. This delightful piece features two human figures cradling a tiny house in their hands. The figures have roots for feet, and green leaves growing from their heads. This was another winner of the Lloyd art competition.

▸Continue straight down the walkway, crossing Weidler and Halsey.

▸Enter Lloyd Center. You are on the mall's second (middle) level. Go straight to the center of the mall. The food court can be found on the third level.

▸Stop at the railing and look down to get a good view of skaters whirling around on the year-round ice rink. Then look up to see the third-level food court with a huge sculpture of bronze birds hanging underneath the dome. *Flight,* by Portland artist Tom Hardy, was commissioned when the Lloyd Center originally opened. This flock of geese now flies above the food court on the third level of the mall. Then take the escalator or elevator down to the first level.

▸Continue straight ahead toward Macy's, and turn right after the ice rink, to Nordstrom. The exit to Multnomah and 9th is to the left just before this store. Go through the exit doors, and you will be back at your starting point.

Walk 20: Beverly Cleary's Neighborhood

✗ 🛒 👫 🏢 ♿

General location: Northeast Portland, about 2 miles east of the Convention Center, in the neighborhoods known as Hollywood and Laurelhurst

Special attractions: If you or your children love Beverly Cleary's children's books, you will all enjoy walking through the Hollywood neighborhood, which was the setting for many of them. This walk also includes neighboring Laurelhurst, a lovely residential area of early-twentieth-century homes. You will pass a small lake in Laurelhurst Park.

Difficulty: Easy; entirely on sidewalk. There is one noticeable hill and a ramped climb on the pedestrian walkway over the freeway; otherwise, the route is flat.

Distance: 7 miles, but the walk may be divided in two

Estimated time: 4 hours for the entire 7 miles

Services: Restaurants can be found in the commercial area around Hancock and 40th Avenue. There are restrooms in Grant Park, at the Hollywood MAX station, and in Laurelhurst Park.

Restrictions: Since these are old neighborhoods, overgrown trees and bushes crowd many sidewalks. Because there are places without curb cuts, the walk is not suitable for wheelchairs. Strollers are fine. No swimming or wading is allowed in the lake in Laurelhurst Park.

For more information: Contact Portland Parks and Recreation or the Multnomah County Library.

Getting started: From I-84 (eastbound), take the NE 33rd Avenue exit. (Westbound traffic exits at 43rd Avenue.) Turn left (north), and cross Broadway and then Schuyler Street.

Public transportation: The MAX light-rail stops at the Hollywood Transit Center. You can take Bus 10 (NE 33rd Avenue) from there to the Grant Park playground.

Overview: Beverly Cleary has been writing award-winning children's books since the 1950s. Cleary used the Hollywood neighborhood, where she grew up, as the setting for her books about Beezus and Ramona Quimby, Henry Huggins, Ellen Tebbits, and Otis Spofford. The neighborhood has not changed much. You will walk by Cleary's childhood homes and see some of the schools, parks, and other places that are named in her books. Cleary also set a few scenes in the Laurelhurst neighborhood, which is directly to the south on the other side of the freeway.

You'll pass some elegant old homes on streets curving around a central traffic circle, and specially designed gates that originally separated the residences from their more-mundane surroundings. The developers were influenced by the "City Beautiful" ideas that became popular after the 1893 World's Fair and Columbian Exhibition in Chicago. Developers had already created an upscale Laurelhurst subdivision in Seattle and wanted to establish the same kind of neighborhood in Portland. The Olmsted Brothers firm of landscape architects planned the park, and it became known as one of the loveliest on the West Coast.

The Walk

▶Begin this walk at the NE 33rd Avenue and Hancock Street MAX #73 bus stop in front of the Beverly Cleary

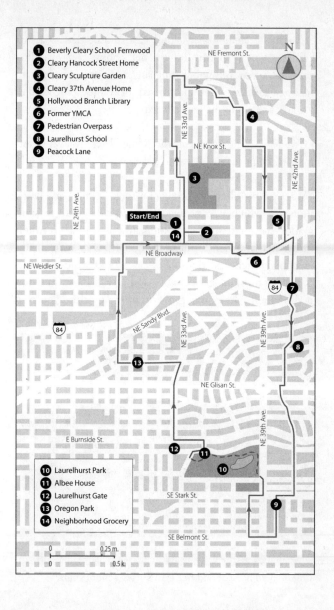

1. Beverly Cleary School Fernwood
2. Cleary Hancock Street Home
3. Cleary Sculpture Garden
4. Cleary 37th Avenue Home
5. Hollywood Branch Library
6. Former YMCA
7. Pedestrian Overpass
8. Laurelhurst School
9. Peacock Lane

10. Laurelhurst Park
11. Albee House
12. Laurelhurst Gate
13. Oregon Park
14. Neighborhood Grocery

N

NE Fremont St.

NE 33rd Ave.

NE Knox St.

NE 42nd Ave.

NE 24th Ave.

Start/End

NE Broadway

NE Weidler St.

84

NE Sandy Blvd.

NE 33rd Ave.

84

NE 39th Ave.

NE 39th Ave.

NE Glisan St.

E Burnside St.

SE Stark St.

SE Belmont St.

0   0.25 m.

0   0.5 k.

School, the elementary school Cleary attended as a first grader, named "Glenwood" in her books. Her own first year there was miserable, but she compensated for it in *Ramona the Pest,* when she created for Ramona the kind of teacher she would have preferred.

▸Cross NE 33rd Avenue at the signal. There is a walk button on the post.

▸Walk half a block to 3340 Hancock Street. This is the house in which Cleary lived from fourth grade to sixth grade. The Craftsman-style bungalow is similar to others in the neighborhood, but every house has its own distinguishing touches in doorways, eaves, and windows. This is still a family neighborhood, and it still looks much as it did when Cleary was growing up. (Any time you read

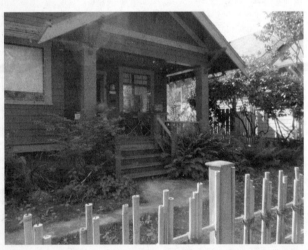

Cleary lived here during her elementary school years.

about something happening on Klickitat Street, this is where it happened; Cleary liked the name Klickitat better than Hancock.) As you walk, you can imagine Henry, Beezus, and Ramona riding past you on their bikes and jumping rope in the driveways.

▶Return to NE 33rd Avenue and turn right, crossing Hancock. Proceed north for two blocks, crossing Tillamook Street and U. S. Grant Place. This was a popular street for drag racers in the 1950s, so it was one of the first in the city to have planters installed in its middle to slow down the traffic.

▶You are at the south end of Grant Park, named for Ulysses S. Grant. Continue north on NE 33rd Avenue along the west side of the park. This is the park in which Henry Huggins dug up night crawlers to sell so that he could reimburse a friend for his lost football. Note the many examples of English cottages on the other side of NE 33rd. Shingled roofs designed to imitate thatched roofs make them easily recognizable. Small arched windows under the eaves display tiny balconies suitable for fairytale princesses, and the main windows are often trimmed with beautiful beveled glass.

Across the park to your right you can see Cleary's alma mater, Ulysses S. Grant High School. Cleary worked on the school newspaper here, and wrote a script for a Girls League play. Her teachers chose Cleary to star in the show. Cleary referred to it as Zachary Taylor High School in her books. The school may look familiar to you because the title character in *Mr. Holland's Opus* was based on a former band teacher at Grant High. The movie was filmed here.

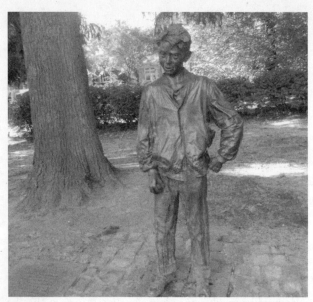

Henry Huggins is one of the statues in the Cleary Sculpture Garden.

▸Just past the street sign for NE Thompson Street, take the blacktop walkway on your right into the park; then take the first path to your left. The bronze figures ahead of you are part of the Beverly Cleary Sculpture Garden.

THE BEVERLY CLEARY SCULPTURE GARDEN

The Friends of Henry and Ramona, a volunteer group of teachers, librarians, neighbors, and businesspeople, built this garden. It was funded by donations from Cleary fans throughout the United States and Canada.

Portland artist Lee Hunt created these life-size figures of Ribsy, Henry, and Ramona. She used real 1950s clothing on wax models to get the right textures. Ramona, in new boots and flying raincoat, gaily splashes in the fountain. Henry, with a Band-Aid on one hand and an apple bulging from the pocket of his oddly fastened jacket, looks bemused. Ribsy seems surprised at water squirting between his paws. One

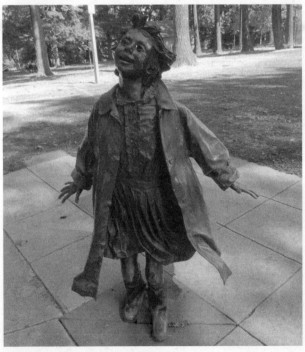

Ramona frolics in her new boots.

neighborhood resident claims she's seen dogs trying to rub noses with the statue of Ribsy.

Take time to read the titles of Cleary's books etched in the red granite stones surrounding the fountain.

▶Exit the sculpture garden by the figure of Ribsy and take the path back to the walkway. Turn right, and go down the steps to NE 33rd Avenue.

▶Cross NE 33rd at the crosswalk carefully, as there are no signals here.

▶Go straight ahead on NE Brazee Street for one block, to 32nd Place.

▶Turn right onto 32nd Place, cross NE Brazee, and continue north for four blocks to NE Klickitat Street.

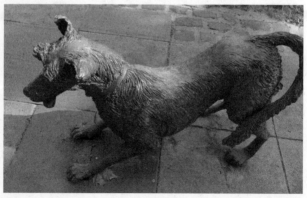

Ribsy's been known to fool real dogs.

▶Cross NE Klickitat and turn right, and walk up the hill for one block to NE 33rd Avenue.

▶Look up to your left. You are halfway up the NE 33rd Avenue Hill. This street used to be closed to traffic when it snowed, and Henry Huggins liked to slide down it on his Flexible Flyer sled. It's steep enough that locals called it "Dead Man's Hill."

▶Cross NE 33rd at the pedestrian light. Turn right. Go one block to NE Siskiyou Street, cross, and turn left.

▶Cross NE 34th and NE 35th Avenues and follow the sidewalk that curves to the right. Take the first left, and you will still be on Siskiyou Street. Continue to NE 36th Avenue.

▶Turn right at NE 36th Avenue and go to NE Morris. Turn left, crossing NE 36th.

▶Continue one block to NE 37th. Cross NE Morris and NE 37th, then turn right.

▶Find 2924 NE 37th Avenue, on the east side of the street. Cleary moved to this tan house with brown trim when she was in sixth grade. She chose the front bedroom for her own, feeling it would put greater distance between her and her parents in their back bedroom. Her father bought her a bike so she could get back and forth to Fernwood (now Beverly Cleary) School.

Cleary's best friend, Claudine Klum, lived only a block away. Claudine was the inspiration for Austine in Cleary's book, *Ellen Tebbits,* and her house was the model for the Huggins family home.

▸Continue on NE 37th, crossing Stanton to Knott Street.

▸Cross Knott Street and turn left. Henry Huggins got four kittens at a rummage sale on his way to Knott Street. This was where *Oregon Journal* papers were delivered, and Henry wanted to ask Mr. Capper for a job as a paperboy. He hid the kittens in his jacket during the interview.

▸Turn right onto Cesar Chavez (39th) Avenue and continue three blocks south to Tillamook Street. Turn left. The Hollywood shopping district begins at Tillamook Street. You can find small coffee bars and restaurants in

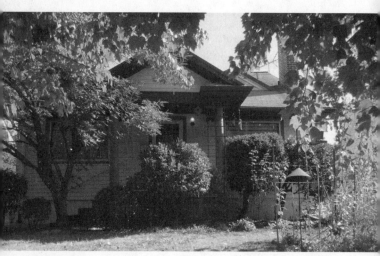

Cleary moved to 2924 37th Avenue when she was in sixth grade.

this area. Ellen Tebbits, the main character in the book of the same name, lived near Tillamook and 41st Avenue.

▶Continue two more blocks to NE 41st Avenue. Cross Tillamook to the entrance of the Hollywood branch of the Multnomah County Library. This is such a reading neighborhood that there have been two replacements for the original Rose City Library Carnegie library building Beverly Cleary used. The librarians will be happy to give you more information about Mrs. Cleary.

Cleary decided to pursue a career as a writer after winning a $2 first prize in an essay contest. Later, she found out that no one else had entered. Her mother argued that she would need a more reliable way to earn a living. Because the Rose City Library was Cleary's favorite refuge, she became a librarian before she began writing stories.

▶Exit the library at the corner of 41st Avenue.

▶Cross 41st and turn right. Walk two blocks, passing the Rite Aid Pharmacy, the model for the Colossal Drugstore in Cleary's books. In *Otis Spofford,* the Spofford School of Dance is located over this drugstore.

▶Stop at Sandy Boulevard. From here you can see the Hollywood Theater, an exuberant example of the Art Deco style. It stands on the other side of Sandy, between 41st and 42nd Avenues. It was considered one of Portland's most magnificent theaters when it was built in 1926. In the days of silent movies, the organist and Wurlitzer organ rose slowly on a platform from the basement. The theater

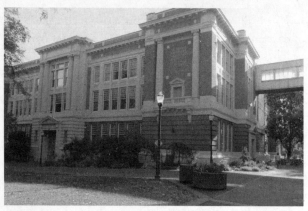

This is Fernwood, Cleary's elementary school.

was so well known that it gave its name to this district, originally known as Rose City Park.

(Author's Note: You have now gone 2 miles. If you wish to return to your starting point, follow the directions below. You then will have walked nearly 3 miles. If you wish to walk more of Cleary's neighborhood, follow the directions on page 233 for the Laurelhurst Loop.)

▶To return to your starting point, veer right on Sandy, and go two blocks to Broadway.

▶Turn right onto Broadway, and go west to 38th Avenue. Just south of this corner, at 1630 NE 38th, is the Northeast Community Center, once the YMCA where Henry Huggins swam in its indoor pool.

▶Cross 38th and continue on Broadway for two blocks to 36th Avenue.

▸Turn right on 36th. Go one block north to Schuyler Street.

▸Turn left and continue west for two long blocks on Schuyler to NE 33rd Avenue.

▸Turn right on NE 33rd.

▸Continue one block to Hancock. Cross NE 33rd at the signal. Turn by the grocery store parking lot.

Laurelhurst Loop

▸Cross Sandy Boulevard and turn left. Continue for one block to 41st Place. Turn right onto the alleyway, 41st Place.

▸Proceed on 42nd Avenue, crossing Broadway, Weidler, and Halsey Streets. Look for the pedestrian overpass signs.

▸Look for the pedestrian steps straight ahead. Ramps to the overpass are to the right. Go up and over the freeway and down the other side to Senate Street. You are now in the Laurelhurst neighborhood. This neighborhood with its curvilinear streets was inspired by the "City Beautiful" ideas from Chicago's Columbian Exposition.

▸Continue south on 42nd Avenue, located at the base of the steps. (If you used the ramp, return to the steps.)

▸Cross Multnomah and then Hassalo Street at the crosswalk, then cross Hazelfern Place to Laurelhurst Place.

Cross 42nd to Laurelhurst School. This school was the inspiration for Cedarhurst School in *Ramona Quimby, Age 8*. Ramona started third grade here with teacher Mrs. Whaley, and became friends with "Yard Ape." Return to the west side of 42nd.

▶As you cross Royal Court and continue south, you will notice 42nd Avenue has become 41st. Look to the right at Glisan, and you can see the shiny gold statue of Joan of Arc. It centers the very busy Coe Circle.

▶Stay on 41st and cross Glisan at the pedestrian signal. Continue south for four more blocks to NE Burnside.

▶Cross Burnside at the signal and continue for five more blocks, to Stark Street. The street signs have change to SE. Cross Stark carefully, as there are no signals here.

▶Turn right for about a block until you see the sign for Peacock Lane. Turn left and proceed on the west side of Peacock Lane. This unique, well-kept, English-style neighborhood was an early subdivision. Developer R. F. Wassell used a similar design for these five- to seven-room houses and incorporated the best street lighting available at the time. Builders bought materials in large quantities and constructed several houses at once.

Each house has distinguishing windows and entryways. This combination of quality touches and cookie-cutter styles makes Peacock Lane unique. You can see strings of lights hanging on most of the houses. The area is well known for its decorations at Christmastime.

▶Peacock Lane ends at Belmont Street. Turn right onto Belmont for one block, cross Cesar Chavez Avenue, and continue to 38th Avenue.

▶Turn north on 38th for four blocks, to Stark Street.

▶Turn right onto Stark to the sidewalk along 39th (Cesar Chavez) Avenue. Turn left and cross. Proceed north, crossing Oak, and enter Laurelhurst Park. This 25-acre park, including its lake, was designed by a Portland Parks superintendent, Emanuel Mische, who had been a horticulturist in the Olmsted Brothers' landscape firm.

▶At the Y, take the path that bends right to the small spring-fed lake with its resident population of turtles, fish, and ducks. It occasionally freezes over and becomes a good place for ice skating. Otis Spofford and Ellen Tebbits skated here in two of Cleary's books.

This is obviously a well-loved park where people jog, stroll, and walk dogs. Tall, old trees shade benches and picnic tables. Volunteers maintain all park flower beds. There are a horseshoe pit, playgrounds, and courts for tennis, volleyball, and basketball.

▶Facing the pond, walk to the right. Take the asphalt path on the walk to the left around the west end of the pond, and then take the asphalt path on the left toward the restrooms. Continue straight past the restrooms and picnic areas. Veer at the Y near the northwest corner of the park to exit the park at 33rd Avenue.

▶Turn right onto Ankeny and continue past lovely estate homes until you see the sign for Floral Place. You are standing in front of 3360 Ankeny, a 6,900-square-foot brick Colonial Revival building designed by Portland's famous architect, A. E. Doyle, for an early Portland mayor named H. Russell Albee. The house and 0.75-acre lot have a great view of the park, which is fitting, since Albee became a leading advocate of Portland's park system.

▶Turn left and cross Ankeny, keeping on the left side of Floral Place.

▶Continue straight for one block, to Burnside.

▶Turn left onto Burnside Street and walk to 32nd Avenue (a continuation of 33rd Avenue). Notice the Laurelhurst gate at this intersection. These gates were designed to separate residential Laurelhurst from the surrounding commercial district.

▶Cross Burnside at the signal.

▶Stay on NE 32nd to Glisan Street, where you can see another Laurelhurst gate.

▶Look for the push buttons that control the signals. Cross Glisan and 32nd with the lights. On your left is the Greek Orthodox Church of the Holy Trinity.

▶Continue north on 32nd, past this church. Cross Hoyt Street, and continue one block to Irving Street.

▶Turn left (west) onto Irving for two blocks. When you cross 30th, you will find yourself in Oregon Park. This small neighborhood park is a nice place for children to play.

▶Continue straight through the park. Exit on Irving Street and continue one more block to 28th.

▶Turn right onto 28th and walk two blocks to Sandy Boulevard.

▶Cross Sandy at the walk signal—there is a push button— and continue north to Holladay. The bridge over the freeway is straight ahead. Cleary lived on Halsey Street next to Sullivan's Gulch, the name for the canyon where the freeway is located today. Ben Holladay used this gulch for Oregon's first railroad.

▶Cross the freeway and continue straight on the wide sidewalk.

▶Keep heading north. After you cross Wasco Street, you can see the new Hollywood West Fred Meyer store on the right. There are restrooms and a deli inside the store.

▶Cross Clackamas. The sidewalk jogs to the right at Halsey Street. A nice little park is situated here, at the Weidler end of the Fred Meyer parking lot.

▶Cross Weidler and Broadway. Continue one block and turn right on Schuyler.

▸Continue (east) for two blocks. Just before you reach NE 33rd Avenue, cross Schuyler. The grocery store on your left was once Kienow's grocery and dime store. Beverly Cleary used this parking lot as the setting for several incidents in her books. In *Ramona the Pest,* Ramona lost her brand-new boots when she got stuck in the mud during the store's construction. She picked burrs here to make a crown for her head in *Ramona and Her Father,* when she got bored waiting for her father to finish meeting with her teacher. This is also where Henry's dog, Ribsy, got a parking ticket in *Henry and Beezus.*

▸Cross Hancock to your starting place in front of the Beverly Cleary Middle School.

Walk 21: The Grotto

📷 ✕ 🏢 ♿

General location: Northeast Portland, 3 miles south of Portland International Airport

Special attractions: Gardens, statuary (including a replica of Michelangelo's Pietà, chapels, gift shop, and a spectacular view north across the Columbia River

Difficulty: Easy walk on paved paths, with an elevator to the upper gardens

Distance: 1 mile, including walks on both levels

Estimated time: 2 hours

Services: A coffee bar, gift shop, and wheelchair-accessible restrooms are available at the Welcome Center.

Restrictions: A $4 token must be purchased at the Welcome Center or the Visitor Complex to gain access to the upper level of gardens. The Grotto is open daily except on Thanksgiving and Christmas. No pets are permitted.

For more information: Contact the Grotto.

Getting started: From I-205 northbound, take the Sandy Boulevard West exit to NE 85th Avenue. Follow the signs to the Grotto entrance.

Public transportation: Bus 12 (Sandy) stops at the entrance to the Grotto. Contact TriMet for information about fares and schedules (trimet.org).

Overview: Only five minutes from Portland International Airport, this 62-acre Roman Catholic sanctuary, founded by the Servites, is a peaceful retreat from the bustle of modern life. Take a leisurely stroll through the woodsy plaza level, where vines and shrubs muffle the noise of nearby

Sandy Boulevard, and admire the replica of Michelangelo's *Pietà* inside a rock grotto. An elevator lifts you to the top of a 110-foot cliff. At the top, you'll find incredible views and beautifully manicured gardens. Mr. Butchart, known for the Butchart Gardens on Vancouver Island, donated plants from his gardens and helped with the layout of the grounds.

Statues are everywhere, many of them carved in Italy from Carrara marble.

The Welcome Center contains a gift shop and coffee bar, and the Visitor Complex displays and sells Nativity sets from all over the world. Special religious and musical events often take place on these grounds, including a December "Christmas Festival of Lights."

THE GROTTO

When Ambrose Mayer was a small boy in Canada, he prayed for his mother's recovery from a difficult childbirth and promised he would one day do a great work for the Catholic Church. His mother recovered, and Ambrose kept his promise. This beautiful and peaceful place is the result.

He joined the Order of Servants of Mary (Servites), and, in 1918, was sent as their first pastor to Portland. He bought this former quarry, and a cave was carved out of the 110-foot basalt cliff. The stone was used for the large altar in front of the Grotto. A replica of Michelangelo's *Pietà* was installed. Ever since it was named a national sanctuary in 1983, it has provided a peaceful haven to visitors of all faiths.

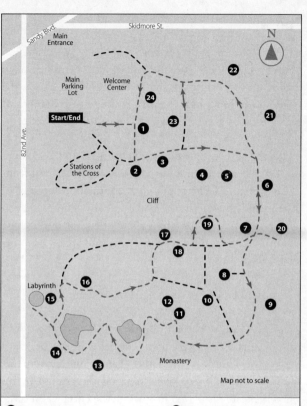

1 Clotilde Merio Plaza

2 Sacred Heart Statue

3 St. Philip Benizi Statue

4 The Grotto Cave with *Pietà* and Main Alter

5 St. Peregrine Shrine

6 Elevator to Upper Level Gardens

7 Meyer Memorial Garden Plaza

8 Saint Jude Thaddeus Statue

9 Saint Joseph's Grove

10 Chapel of St. Anne

11 Assumption of Mary Statue and Rose Garden

12 Peace Pole

13 Marguerite M. Casey Peace Garden

14 Glorious Mysteries

15 Luminous Mysteries

16 The Way of Our Sorrowful Mother

17 Lithuanian Wayside Shrine

18 St. Francis of Assisi Statue

19 Statue of Our Sorrowful Mother

20 Meditation Chapel

21 Chapel of Mary

22 Visitor Complex

23 Christus Garden

24 Madonna of Orvieto

The Walk

▶The walk begins at the parking lot at Sandy Boulevard and 85th Avenue. As you enter the parking lot, a beautiful Italian marble Calvary tableau at the south end of the lot sets the stage. Just beyond, near the path leading to the Stations of the Cross, is a bas-relief plaque of President John F. Kennedy.

▶Take the path leading directly to the plaza and stop at the display case on the Clotilde Merlo Plaza, directly in front of the Welcome Center. This gives information about what is here, and where. The Welcome Center will provide you with a map and information about the Grotto. Purchase elevator tokens at the gift shop. Restrooms are located outside the building.

▶Turn right and go to the *Sacred Heart* statue.

▶Take the path to the left. On the hill to your right, next to a stream, is a marble statue of Saint Philip Benizi, a Servite, who hid in a cave rather than being elected pope. He is kneeling, with a papal tiara on the ground by his side. The statue is placed just before the entrance into the main plaza.

▶Descend into the main plaza for a full view of the Grotto, a cave carved from the cliff, with two candle-bearing angels on either side of the replica of Michelangelo's *Pietà*. Racks of votive candles flank the altar in front of the cave, and recordings of Gregorian chants float through the area. Mass is celebrated here every Sunday at noon during the summer months.

▶At the left edge of the altar area is a mosaic icon of Saint Peregrine Laziosi, the patron saint of those suffering from life-threatening diseases. The leg sores of this thirteenth-century Servite brother were miraculously cured through prayer the night before his leg was to be amputated.

▶The tall concrete structure housing the elevator is south of the Grotto plaza, against the 110-foot cliff on your right. Take the path leading to it, drop your token in the turnstile, and enter the elevator.

When it arrives at the cliff top, the elevator doors open onto the Meyer Memorial Garden Plaza. Restrooms can be found to your left. Signs pointing to the Upper Gardens are directly in front of you.

▶Enter the main gardens. On your right, you will see a directory and map. Note the many small pathways leading to various statues and shrines. If you explore any of these, return to the main walkway after your visit.

▶Take the walkway to your left, passing a small path on the right that leads to the statue of Saint Jude Thaddeus.

▶The main walk goes by the large trees marking Saint Joseph's Grove. Bas-relief panels, depicting both the joys and sorrows of his life, are on either side of Saint Joseph's statue. The next path to your right leads to the charming Chapel of Saint Anne in a lovely garden.

▶Continue on the main walkway, past the Servite Monastery that houses the priests and brothers who staff the

Grotto. Neither this building nor the convent in the rear is open to the public. In front of the monastery is the statue of the Assumption of Mary, surrounded by a rose garden. Walk around the garden to the opposite side, admiring the rose bushes donated by the Royal Rosarians, a group of active civic leaders. The plaque at the base of the fountain honors their deceased members.

▶The statue faces the walkway to the Peace Pole, dedicated in 1988 to prayer for world peace. Take this walk to your left and read the message—MAY PEACE PREVAIL ON EARTH—inscribed in English, Japanese, Russian, and Spanish.

▶Continue past a reflection pond to the Marguerite M. Casey Peace Garden, where you will find the first of four plaques by Oregon artist Mary Lewis. This one depicts the *Joyful Mystery of the Rosary*. Follow the walkway passing one

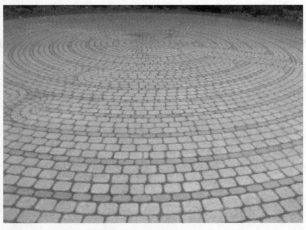

Walking a labyrinth brings about a sense of peace.

for the *Sorrowful Mystery*. The sound and sight of waterfalls and flowing water enhance the serene garden setting as you view another pond, and then go by the plaque for the *Glorious Mystery*. A side path here leads you into a labyrinth, modeled after one at Chartres Cathedral in France.

▶Return to the walkway passing Mary Lewis's fourth plaque, for the *Luminous Mysteries*. A path to your left leads to the Filipino Faith shrine. Take the main walk to the right along the *Way of Our Sorrowful Mother*, passing glass cases with scenes representing painful events in Mary's life. The thirty-four life-size figures, carved from white pine by Professor Heider of Pietralba, Italy, are considered some of the loveliest woodcarvings in the United States.

▶After viewing the last station, keep on the main walkway past the ancient Lithuanian wayside shrine on your left. This gift from Portland and Chicago Lithuanians combines both pagan symbols of tree worship and those symbolizing Christianity.

Around some bushes on your right is a bronze Saint Francis of Assisi with animal friends; it was created by local artist Michael Florin Dente, and dedicated in 1993.

▶Ahead on your left, high on a stone pillar, is the statue of *Our Sorrowful Mother*. Walk to the north side and look up to see Mary, depicted as standing at the foot of the Cross and hearing Jesus tell John to now consider her to be his mother.

▶Cross to the green iron fence to see a magnificent vista of the mountains and Columbia River. You can see Mount

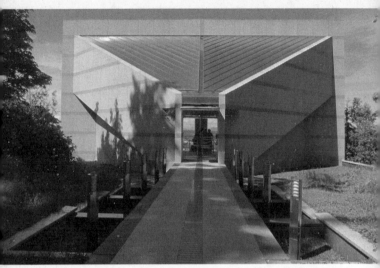

The Meditation Chapel is aptly named.

St. Helens, Mount Adams, and sometimes Mount Rainier from this viewpoint near the cliff's edge.

▶Return to the walkway that leads you back into the Meyer Plaza. Instead of taking the elevator down, cross the plaza and take the walkway leading to the stunning Marilyn Moyer Meditation Chapel. A raised walkway leads to the entrance. You will be struck immediately by the awe-inspiring view through the beveled-glass bow window, once featured in *Architecture* magazine. This window is a work of art in itself, and offers one of the best 180-degree views in the Portland area, from the airport to Mount St. Helens. Centered in front of this window is a rare bronze cast of Michelangelo's *Pietà*. The simply furnished chapel provides a perfect setting for meditation.

▶Return to the elevator and descend to the lower level. After you exit, turn right to visit the Chapel of Mary on the east side of the Main Plaza. Daily Mass is celebrated in this beautiful marble sanctuary. Soft light filters from the 25-foot-high stained-glass window celebrating the Resurrection. Spanish-born José De Soto, an artist who painted movie sets, created the murals.

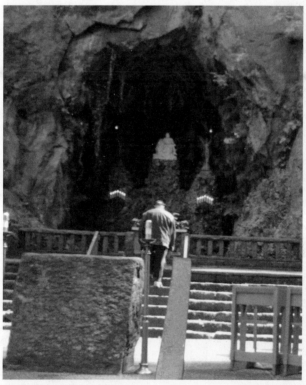

A copy of Michelangelo's *Pietà* resides in the Meditation Chapel.

▸As you leave the chapel, turn right to the Visitor Complex, staffed with knowledgeable volunteers who can answer almost any question you may have about the Grotto. The gift shop contains a small display of art and an exceptionally large collection of Nativity sets. Created in a wide variety of sizes, and reflecting the country of origin, these are available for purchase. A conference center available for groups of up to 225 people is on the lower level.

▸Leave the Visitor Center, turn right, and pass the security building. Restrooms are located in the lower level of this building.

▸Turn left and skirt the west side of the plaza, following the signs to the Christus Garden. Within a rhododendron grove is a bronze statue of Christ carrying his cross to Calvary.

▸Turn back to the main walkway, turning left to the large glass case with the *Madonna of Orvieto.* This revolving artwork is based on a painting in Orvieto, Italy. The four two-sided panels rotate, with the colored sides showing the Madonna, and the white sides depicting marble carvings similar to those found in the same church.

▸Return to the Clotilde Merlo Plaza. Take the walkway by the Welcome Center back to your starting point in the parking lot, or take the path on your left to the Stations of the Cross path, which will also lead you back to the parking lot, where Station 1 is located.

Walk 22: East Airport Way

✕ 🛒 🏢 ♿

General location: Just east of I-205 and Portland International Airport

Special attractions: A chance to stretch your legs and enjoy a bit of the natural Columbia Slough in the midst of the airport-motel district

Difficulty: Easy, flat, entirely on sidewalks with curb cuts; wheelchair-accessible

Distance: 1.5 miles

Estimated time: 30 minutes

Services: There are restaurants, restrooms, and water available at the motels.

Restrictions: None.

For more information: Ask at the reception desks of any of the motels on Airport Way, including the Marriott Courtyard, Fairfield Inn, Holiday Inn Express, Shilo Inn, Clarion, Comfort Suites, and Staybridge Suites.

Getting started: Take Airport Way East underneath I-205 to the junction with Glenn Widing Drive. You will see motels on both sides of the road.

Public transportation: Bus 12 (Sandy) stops on 82nd near the Marriott Courtyard and at the airport. The MAX train also runs to the airport. Contact TriMet for information about fares and schedules (trimet.org).

If you have a long layover between flights, it is possible to take this walk by taking a shuttle bus to one of the motels. Construction at the airport means that pickup stops can

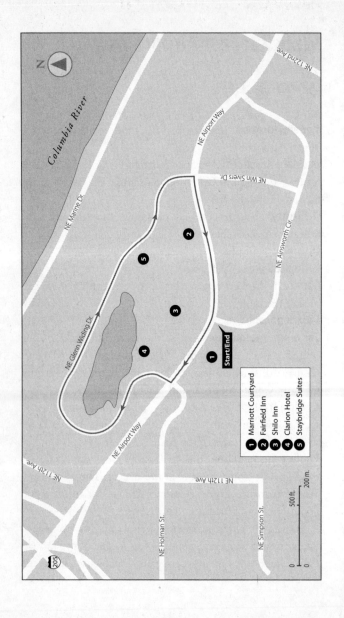

change, so check with the guides at the airport and follow signs to the designated area for buses and shuttles.

Overview: This area recently has become a motel and commercial district serving the Portland International Airport. A small pond still remains in the center of the area; it is part of the Columbia River Slough, which the Port of Portland is maintaining as open space, even as development goes on all around it. These sloughs are important watersheds, providing homes to many types of wildlife, as well as a pleasant respite from the commotion of the airport and motels.

The Walk

▶Begin this walk from any of the motels on Airport Way East. Take the sidewalk on the north side of the road and walk west toward the junction with Glenn Widing Drive. Turn right on the concrete sidewalk.

▶Pass the Clarion Motel. On your right is a small natural pond, part of the Columbia River Slough. It is bordered by brush, cattails, willows, and evergreens. Red-winged blackbirds enjoy these environs, and you may even see Portland's official bird, the great blue heron, fishing for dinner.

▶Stay on the sidewalk as it turns to the right, following Glenn Widing Drive. The road can be busy at times, with commercial ventures on the north side attracting shoppers, but the south side has been preserved as a natural area. As the walk turns east on the north side of the pond, you should have a good view of Mount Hood. Look across a small meadow on your right for another view of the pond.

This area used to be private property, and you can see the remnants of once-cultivated plants bordering the property. In another meadow you can see the remains of a beaver-chewed tree. Now cottontail rabbits enjoy the habitat as it reverts back to a natural state.

▶You get another glimpse of the pond on your right, just before the driveway to the Staybridge Suites. On your left is the International Corporate Center. It adjoins the Airport Way Corporate Park as it meets Airport Way East.

▶Continue past the Staybridge Suites driveway. The next driveway on your right belongs to the Fairfield Inn. You can cut through their parking lot to Airport Way East or stay on the sidewalk. Continue east toward the airport, passing the Shilo Inn on your way to the junction with Glenn Widing Drive.

Appendix A: Other Sights

You may enjoy several other attractions in Portland, or nearby. They may not involve much walking, but they have been enjoyed by visitors and Oregonians of all ages.

Hiking

The Columbia Gorge begins in Troutdale, 12 miles east of Portland. It has wonderful waterfalls, gorgeous views, and hiking trails suited to all abilities. Take I-84 eastbound to exit 35 to access the old Columbia Gorge Scenic Highway. This route passes Vista House at Crown Point, which offers an unusual and spectacular view of the Columbia River, along with tourist information and gifts. It continues on to Multnomah Falls, where you will have a beautiful view of the falls. The lodge has a dining room, snack bar, and a gift store. Ask in the lodge for information about the trail's reopening, as well as information about other nearby trails.

Museums (all in Portland)

Architectural Heritage Center
701 SE Grand Avenue
(503) 231-7264
visitahc.org

The Hat Museum
1928 SE Ladd Avenue
(503) 232-0433
thehatmuseum.com

Oregon Museum of Science and Industry (OMSI)
1945 SE Water Avenue
(503) 797-4000
omsi.edu

Portland Children's Museum
4015 SW Canyon Road
(503) 223-6500
portlandcm.org
Adults are not permitted without children. There are activities for all ages designed to stretch imagination and knowledge.

Appendix B: Contact Information

Throughout this book we have advised you to contact local attractions, museums, and shops to confirm opening times, locations, and entrance fees. The list below gives you the phone numbers and addresses of places mentioned. These are also repeated in the walk listings.

Oregon Convention Center
777 NE Martin Luther King Jr. Boulevard
(503) 235-7575
(800) 791-2250
oregoncc.org

Portland Oregon Visitors Association
701 SW 6th Avenue
(503) 275-8355
travelportland.com
The Portland Oregon Visitors Association has a wealth of information about Portland. If you are in town, stop by the Visitor Center or call them with your questions.

Activities, Attractions, and Museums
The Friends of Mount Tabor
taborfriends.com

The Grotto
8840 NE Skidmore Street
Portland 97220
(503) 254-7371
thegrotto.org

Hoyt Arboretum
4000 SW Fairview Boulevard
(503) 865-8733
hoytarboretum.org

Japanese Gardens
611 SW Kingston Avenue
(503) 223-1321
japanesegarden.com

Oregon History Center
1200 SW Park Avenue
(503) 222-1741
ohs.org

Oregon Maritime Museum
113 SW Naito Parkway
(503) 224-7724
oregonmaritimemuseum.org

Oregon Museum of Science and Industry (OMSI)
1945 SE Water Avenue
(503) 797-4000
omsi.edu

Oregon Zoo
4001 SW Canyon Road
(503) 226-1561
oregonzoo.org

Portland Audubon Society and Nature Store
5151 NW Cornell Road
(503) 292-9453
audubonportland.com

Portland Center for the Performing Arts
1111 SW Broadway
(503) 248-4336
pcpa.com

Portland Parks and Recreation
1120 SW 5th Avenue, Suite 1302
(503) 823-7529
portlandoregon.gov/parks

Portland Police Museum
1111 SW 2nd Avenue
(503) 823-0019
portlandpolicemuseum.com

World Forestry Center
4033 SW Canyon Road
(503) 228-1367
worldforestry.org

Airport Hotels
Clarion Hotel Airport
11518 Glenn Widing Drive
(503) 252-2222
(800) 994-7878

Fairfield Inn
11929 NE Airport Way
(503) 253-1400
(800) 228-2800

Marriott Courtyard
11550 NE Airport Way
(503) 252-3200
(800) 321-2211
marriotthotels.com

Shilo Suites Hotel
11707 NE Airport Way
(503) 252-7500
shiloinn.com

Staybridge Suites
11936 Glenn Widing Drive
(503) 262-8888
staybridgesuites.com

Convention Center and Lloyd Center Hotels
Crowne Plaza
1441 NE 2nd Avenue
(503) 233-2401

DoubleTree Portland—Lloyd Center
1000 NE Multnomah Street
(503) 281-6111

Lion and the Rose Victorian Bed and Breakfast
1810 NE 15th Avenue
(503) 287-9245
(800) 955-1647
lionrose.com

Red Lion Portland Inn
1021 NE Grand Avenue
(503) 235-2100

Shilo Inn Rose Garden
1506 NE 2nd Avenue
(503) 736-6300

Downtown Hotels
Ace Hotel
1022 SW Stark Street
(503) 228-2277
acehotel.com/portland

The Benson Hotel
309 SW Broadway
(503) 228-2000
bensonhotel.com

Embassy Suites at the Multnomah Hotel
319 SW Pine Street
(503) 279-9000

The Governor Hotel
614 SW 11th Avenue
(503) 224-3400
governorhotel.com

The Heathman Hotel
1001 SW Broadway
(503) 790-7752
portland.heathmanhotel.com

Hotel deLuxe
729 SW 15th Avenue
(503) 219-2094
hoteldeluxeportland.com

The Mark Spencer Hotel
409 SW 11th Avenue
(503) 224-3293
markspencer.com/

Marriott Hotel—Downtown Waterfront
1401 SW Naito Parkway
(503) 226-7600

The Portland Hilton Hotel
921 SW 6th Avenue
(503) 226-1611

RiverPlace Hotel
1510 SW Harbor Way
(503) 228-3233
riverplacehotel.com

Travelodge
2401 SW 4th Avenue
(503) 226-1122

Colleges and Universities
Lewis and Clark College
0615 SW Palatine Hill Road
(503) 768-7000
lclark.edu

Portland State University
Smith Memorial Student Union, PSU
1825 SW Broadway
(503) 725-3000
pdx.edu

Reed College
3203 SE Woodstock Boulevard
(503) 771-1112
(800) 547-4750
reed.edu

Shopping
Lloyd Center
2201 Lloyd Center (corner of NE 9th and Multnomah)
(503) 282-2511
lloydcenter.com

Portland Pioneer Place
700 SW 5th Avenue
(503) 228-5800
pioneerplace.com

Powell's City of Books
1005 W. Burnside
(503) 228-4651
powells.com

Transportation
Amtrak/Union Station
800 NW 6th Avenue
(503) 273-4866
amtrak.com

Portland Airport
7000 NE Airport Way
(503) 460-4040
portofportland.com

Portland Streetcar
(503) 823-2900
portlandstreetcar.com

TriMet Transportation District of Oregon
1412 SE 17th Avenue
(503) 238-RIDE (7433)
trimet.org
All buses and light-rail transportation services are part of the TriMet system.

Appendix C: Great Tastes

As you walk through Portland, you will notice many small coffee and/or sandwich shops, pubs, and other types of eateries. They can be found along the streets, on the college campuses, and inside the shopping centers.

There are far too many to list in this guide. The Official Visitors Guide, available at the Portland Oregon Visitors Association, lists restaurants by type of food and price. The newspapers frequently have information on the latest openings and closings and reviews, as does the *Portland Monthly* magazine (portlandmonthlymag.com/).

The following list includes some of the major restaurants you will pass while taking the walks listed in this book.

Restaurants

Aquariva
0470 SW Hamilton Cout
(503) 802-5850
aquarivaportland.com

Bambuza Vietnam Bistro
3682 SW Bond Avenue
(503) 206-6330
bambuza.com

Dan & Louis Oyster Bar Restaurant
208 SW Ankeny Street
(503) 227-5906
danandlouis.com

Goose Hollow Inn
1927 SW Jefferson
(503) 228-7010
goosehollowinn.com

Huber's Café
411 SW 3rd Avenue
(503) 228-5686
hubers.com/index.html

Jake's Famous Crawfish
401 SW 12th Avenue
(503) 226-1419
mccormickandschmicks.com/locations/portland-oregon/
portland-oregon/sw12thave.aspx

Jake's Grill at the Governor Hotel
611 SW 10th Avenue
(503) 220-1850
governorhotel.com/dining.html

Lair Hill Bistro
2823 SW 1st Avenue
(503) 279-0200
lairhillbistro.com

The Leaky Roof
16th Avenue and SW Jefferson
(503) 222-3745
theleakyroof.com

McCormick & Schmick's Seafood Restaurant
0309 SW Montgomery Street
(503) 220-1865
mccormickandschmicks.com

Porcelli's Ristorante & Bar
6500 SW Virginia Avenue
(503) 245-2260
porcellisristorante.com

Portland City Grill
111 SW 5th Avenue, 30th Floor
(503) 450-0030
portlandcitygrill.com

Southpark Seafood Grill
901 SW Salmon Street
(503) 326-1300
southparkseafood.com

Stanford's Restaurant at Lloyd Center
913 Lloyd Center (NE corner of 9th and Multnomah)
(503) 335-0811
stanfords.com

Appendix D: Useful Phone Numbers

Emergency Numbers
Poison Control
(503) 494-8968
(800) 222-1222

Portland Fire Bureau
Emergency: 911
Nonemergency: (503) 823-3700

Portland Police Bureau
Emergency: 911
Nonemergency: (503) 230-2121
(503) 243-7575

Hospitals

Northeast Portland
Legacy Emanuel Hospital
2801 N. Gantenbein Avenue
(503) 413-2200

Providence Portland Medical Center
4805 NE Glisan Street
(503) 215-1111

Northwest Portland
Legacy Good Samaritan Hospital and Medical Center
1015 NW 22nd Avenue
(503) 413-7711

Southwest Portland
Oregon Health Sciences University (OHSU)
3181 SW Sam Jackson Park Road
(503) 494-8311

Providence St. Vincent Medical Center
9205 SW Barnes Road
(503) 216-1234

Southeast Portland
Providence Milwaukie Hospital
10150 SE 32nd Avenue
Milwaukie, OR 97222
(503) 513-8300

Newspapers and Magazines
The Oregonian
(503) 221-8240
oregonlive.com

Portland Monthly
921 SW Washington Street, Suite 750
(503) 222-5144
portlandmonthlymag.com

Portland Tribune
6605 SE Lake Road
(503) 226-6397
portlandtribune.com

Willamette Week
(503) 243-2122
wweek.com

Appendix E: Read All About It

Want to learn more about Portland? The Multnomah County Library has a major Portland collection. Call (503) 988-5234, or visit multnomah.lib.or.us.

The following books are but a sample of the many you might enjoy.

Oldies (But Still Interesting)

Bianco, Joe. *Portland Step-by-Step with Joe Bianco: A Walking Guide to Scenic and Historic Points of Interest.* Beaverton, OR: Touchstone Press, 1988.

Klooster, Karl I. *Round the Roses: Portland Past Perspectives.* A Collection of Columns Published in *This Week Magazine* between May 1983 and November 1987. Portland, OR: 1987. (Author's Note: Both Bianco and Klooster are former newspapermen. Bianco shares his knowledge as he walks you through the city. Klooster's book consists of reprints of his offbeat columns about quirky happenings in past and present Portland.)

O'Donnell, Terence, and Thomas Vaughan. *Portland: An Informal History and Guide.* Portland: Oregon Historical Society, 1984. (Author's Note: O'Donnell's graceful prose and thorough research make this an excellent guide to the city.)

Snyder, Eugene. *Early Portland: Stump-Town Triumphant.* Portland, OR: Binford and Mort, 1970.

———. *Portland: Names and Neighborhoods.* Portland, OR: Binford and Mort, 1979.

———. *Portland Potpourri: Art, Fountains and Old Friends.* Portland, OR: Binford and Mort, 1991.

(Author's Note: Snyder's accounts of Portland's history are enjoyable, easy to read, and full of interesting anecdotes.)

More-Recent Books

Comerford, Jane. *A History of Northwest Portland: From the River to the Hills.* Portland, OR: Dragonfly Press, 2011.

Foster, Laura. *Portland City Walks.* Portland, OR: Timber Press, 2008.

———. *Portland Hill Walks.* Portland, OR: Timber Press, 2005.

———. *The Portland Stairs Book.* Portland, OR: Timber Press, 2010.

———. *Walk There: 50 Treks in and around Portland and Vancouver.* Portland, OR: Metro, 2008.

Frommer's Portable Portland. New York: John Wiley & Sons, 2010.

Lansing, Jewel and Fred Beck. *Multnomah.* Corvallis, OR: Oregon State University Press, 2012.

Lansing, Jewel Beck. *Portland.* Corvallis, OR: Oregon State University Press, 2003.

Leflar, Stephen. *A History of South Portland.* Unpublished draft, 2011. (Contact: 503-224-5557.)

Munk, Michael. *The Red Book,* 2nd Edition. Portland, OR: Ooligan Press, Portland State University, 2011.

Oregon Blue Book (biannual). Office of the Secretary of State. (Author's Note: This book contains a myriad of facts and figures about Oregon and Portland, plus some of Oregon's history.)

Prince, Tracy J. *Portland's Goose Hollow.* Mount Pleasant, SC: Arcadia Publishing, 2011.

Fiction for Children (and Adults)

Beverly Cleary has written many children's books set in Portland, and two autobiographies. She gives a good view of everyday life in the city. Her two autobiographies are *A Girl from Yamhill* (New York: Morrow, 1988), and *My Own Two Feet* (New York: Morrow, 1996).

Multnomah County Library sponsors a web page with lots of Cleary information. Cleary's Portland children's books were all published by Morrow between 1950 and 1981. If you are taking children on the Beverly Cleary walk, they will enjoy reading some of her books beforehand. The books are enjoyable at any time, but especially in relation to the walks.

Children's Books by Beverly Cleary

Beezus and Ramona
Ellen Tebbits
Henry and Beezus
Henry and the Clubhouse
Henry and the Paper Route
Henry and Ribsy
Henry Huggins
Otis Spofford
Ramona the Brave
Ramona Forever
Ramona and Her Father
Ramona and Her Mother
Ramona the Pest
Ramona Quimby, Age 8
Ribsy

The Wildwood Chronicles

Colin Meloy of the musical group, the Decemberists, and his illustrator wife, Carson Ellis, have written a series (2011) called *The Wildwood Chronicles,* set in Forest Park (wildwoodchronicles.com). You can compare the maps in their books with a map of Forest Park and see how many places match up, even if the events taking place there are imaginary.

Appendix F: Local Walking Resources

Portland is proud of being a friendly, walkable city. Many government resources are behind the effort. One interesting site is walkscore.com, giving prospective residents a chance to find out about walkable neighborhoods.

The Portland Bureau of Transportation, 1120 Southwest 5th Avenue, #800, Portland, OR 97204, has many resources for walkers of all ages and interests. They provide free large-scale bicycle/walking maps for all sectors of the city, showing the location of drinking fountains and traffic signals. They also sponsor SmartTrips walking programs, such as Ten Toe Express and Senior Strolls. There is also a PedPals link so that seniors (over fifty-five) can meet other walking friends within their neighborhoods. For more information, see the website portlandoregon.gov/transportation.

The American Volkssport Association (AVA) is a network of clubs that sponsor noncompetitive walking, swimming, and hiking events throughout the United States. These walks are usually about 10 kilometers (6.2 miles), and can be done at any time of the year. For more information, check out their website (ava.org), or call the AVA at (210) 659-2112.

The Oregon Trail State Volkswalk Association (OTSVA) is the state chapter of the AVA. For information on all Oregon walking events, contact the OTSVA at P.O. Box 3301, Albany, OR 97321. OTSVA can give you phone numbers for local clubs. Current information on Oregon volkssport events can also be found at walkoregon.org.

Wendy Bumgardner, former secretary of the AVA, has a fine web page (walking.about.com), which includes references to many articles about walking, as well as lists and links to walking all over the world.

Index

About the Author

Sybilla Cook was born in Auburn, New York, and lived in Illinois for twenty-five years before moving to Oregon. Once in Oregon, her love for the outdoors resurfaced, and she began bicycling, hiking, and walking. She has frequently walked the Portland Marathon. She is a former school library media specialist and consultant for schools in Illinois and Oregon, and is the author of many books and articles. She is now working on a biography of children's book illustrators, Berta and Elmer Hader, for the nonprofit Hader Connection.

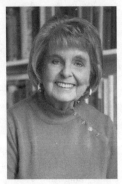

Portrait taken by Colleen Cahill Studios, Portland (colleencahill.com).